Clinical Results of Synovectomy in Rheumatoid Arthritis

Clinical Results of Synovectomy
in Rheumatoid Arthritis

N. GSCHWEND, J. WINER, A. BÖNI, W. BUSSE,
R. DYBOWSKI and J. ZIPPEL;
Kantonsspital Zürich
Universitäts-Rheumaklinik und Institut für physikalische Therapie und
orthopädisch-rheumatologische Klinik Wilhelm Schulthess, Zürich

with 29 figures and 22 tables

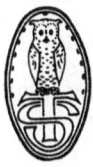

CIP-Kurztitelaufnahme der Deutschen Bibliothek

Gschwend, Norbert
Clinical results of synovectomy in rheumatoid arthritis/
by N. Gschwend; J. Winer; A. Böni —
Darmstadt: Steinkopff, 1977.
    Dt. Ausg. u.d.T.: Gschwend Norbert: Klinische
    Ergebnisse der Synovektomie bei primär
    chronischer Polyarthritis.
    ISBN 978-3-7985-0486-8   ISBN 978-3-642-85924-3 (eBook)
    DOI 10.1007/978-3-642-85924-3
NE: Winer, J.; Böni, Albert

Production: Mono-Satzbetrieb, Darmstadt-Arheilgen

Foreword

In numerous publications the results of synovectomy have been written about where either one or another viewpoint have been examined. In this publication, the attempt is made to collect as many parameters as possible so as to get a most objective picture of the therapeutic worth by studying 100 knee and 370 finger synovectomies.

During the survey, among other points, the following important aspects were taken under consideration:

The operative results were not evaluated by the operating surgeon, but by a rheumatologist who was not on the clinic staff.

As is well known, it is difficult to evaluate the X-ray picture objectively, since very often "subjective impressions" prevail. *Gschwend* succeeded in setting up — mainly for the synovectomized finger joints — a comprehensive point system, so as not to leave the evaluation to chance.

Besides the purely local joint condition, an internal rheumatological status, at the time of the operation and the follow-up examinations, with corresponding laboratory tests, was carried out and included in the evaluation.

Finally, it should be pointed out that this is a long term study of 5 years, with various controls made in between. The examination of so-called control groups, for the present study, seems to us to be highly problematic and of little value for a statement.

Essentially, only the local condition with respect to pain and swellings improves, while the general activity of the inflammatory process as also the mobility and deformity of the synovectomized joints will only be somewhat influenced.

The results of this many-sided study clearly point out the fact that a one-sided therapy tactic, whether this be medication or orthopaedic surgery, can never do justice to the picture of the illness of RA. Only in a well-coordinated team of experts from rheumatology, physical therapy and rehabilitation, as from orthopaedics, can RA-patients be effectively helped. Therefore, synovectomy is not a panacea for the treatment of RA, but can only be incorporated into the total framework of the therapy.

Zürich, Spring 1976   *A. Böni* (Zürich)

CONTENTS

Operative Synovectomy
A critical analysis of the results obtained

1. Historical background

Operative Synovectomy has always been the subject of extremely changing popularity. It will celebrate its 100th birthday in 1977, because *Volkmann* was probably the first perfoming synovectomy on a tuberculous knee joint in 1877. Synovectomy of inflamed rheumatic knee joints became more widespread in Germany at the end of the 19th century *(Schüller, Müller)*, in France *(Mignon)* at the turn of the century and in the USA during the first decades of the twentieth century *(Goldwaith, Murphy)*. The less purposeful selection of patients, a rather traumatizing operation technique and non-systematic after-treatment were probably the major reasons for the somewhat pessimistic assessment of the value of this operation *(Sweet, Ghormley* and *Cameron, Henderson, Allison* and *Coonse, Speed, Jones, Steindler, Boon-Itt)* which more or less fell into oblivion again about twenty years ago.

It was the systematic research of the clinical picture of polyarthritis, the differentiation between its various manifestations, the study of the pathogenesis and pathomorphology of the destruction, as well as the critical assessment of the limited conservative treatment possibilities and chances of success that encouraged the rheumatologists and orthopaedic surgeons in close cooperation *(Laine* and *Vainio, Mason* and *Vaughan-Jackson* etc.) to look for better methods and thus back to the practically forgotten synovectomy.

2. Previous synovectomy papers

It is very difficult to survey the flood of publication that has been written on the subject of synovectomy over the last 15 to 20 years. Nevertheless, both optimism and pessimism are reflected continually between the lines. Is the effort worthwhile for the operated joint, the operated tendon sheet? Is the pathological process influenced in any way? These are only two of the most important questions that still have not been answered definitely.

Table 1. Knee synovectomy—results by various authors.

Authors	Yr. of publ.	number cases	knees	follow-up	stage	surgical procedure	results excellent	good	fair	poor	complications	recurrence
Staf Geens, Clayton, Leidholt, Smyth, Bartholomow	1972	23	31	7–49 months (23 months)	mostly III ARA	synovectomy and débridement	7 42,5%	6	7 28%	11 35,5%		5 cases (biopsy confirmed 2 cases)
Ranawat, Ecker, Straub	1972	46	60	1–8 years (31 months)	II/III ARA	patellectomy 24 ant. and synovectomy 22	1 37%	21	22 37,5%	16 21%	valgus 4 flex. contract. 5 repeat surgerly 16	7 cases
Tillmann	1972		82	6 months–3 years	10 early 72 late synovect.	in late synovect. also menisccctomy (30) removal of osteofyts (34) band replacement (8)	early 6 90% late 33 85	3 28	1 10% 7 9,5%	0 4 5,5%	ligament slackening (7) after addit. surgery	2 cases
Taylor, Harbison, Pepler	1969	78	110	6 months–6 years	II/III/IV ARA	patellectomy 11	60,8%	56 37%	26,8%	37%		
Jakubowski	1972	102	150	2.5–7 yrs.	mostly late synovect.	simple synovect. 91 synovect. + débridement, perhaps patellectomy 59	56 37%	56 37%	38 26%	56 37%	repeat surgery (24) after poor results	
Behnke, Holland	1973	21	32	3 months–3 years (1,7 years)	III (Steinbr.)	débridement 24	9 68,5%	14	3 10,5%	6 21%	ossification of distal quadriceps muscle (1)	
Mohing	1973	140		1–7 years	mostly early synovect.	Mori operation	86,8%		8,7%	4,5%		
Goldie	1974	29	32	7 years	mostly II/III	synovect. and sometimes débridement		24 75%		8 25%	stiffening after synovect. (4)	
Laurin, Derome, Desmarchais, Deziano, Gariepy	1974	49	66	7.5 years	mostly II/III ARA		20 63%	18	13 21,5%	9 15,5%		

Classification — Table 1

Staf Geens, Clayton, Leidholt, Smyth, Bartholomow

excellent	No complaints, improved mobility.
good	No/slight complaints, improved mobility, partial lack of full extension.
fair	Slight pain, swelling same/less, mobility as preoperatively.
poor	Pain, swelling, decrease of ROM.

Ranawat, Ecker, Straub

excellent	No complaints, stable, normal mobility.
good	No complaints, stable, mobility 0—90°.
fair	Occasional pain, mobility as before surgery, lack of full extension.
poor	Pain, unstable, flexion contracture more than 10°.

Taylor, Harbison, Pepler

excellent	No pain, mobility more than 120°.
good	Occasional pain, mobility 90—120°.
fair	Occasional pain, mobility 60—90°.
poor	Intense pain, mobility less than 60°.

Jakubowski

good	No pain or swelling, improvement of mobility.
fair	Occasional pain, mobility as before surgery.
poor	Pain, swelling, decrease of ROM.

Behnke, Holland

excellent	No pain, mobility 0—90°.
good	Occasional pain and swelling, lack of full extension.
fair	Slight pain and swelling, mobility unchanged.
poor	Intense pain, decrease of ROM.

Mohing

good	No/slight complaints, improved/unchanged ROM, improved walking ability.
fair	Less pain, unchanged mobility and walking ability.
poor	Complaints, findings unchanged as before surgery.

Goldie   Own point score.

Laurin, Derome, Desmarchais, Deziano, Gariepy

excellent	No pain, improved mobility.
good	Occasional pain, mobility as before surgery.
fair	Occasional pain, 20% loss of mobility, knee stable.
poor	Pain, knee unstable, 20% or more loss of mobility.

Table 2. Finger synovectomy—results by various authors

Authors	years of publ.	Number		Operated joints	Follow-up	Results				Recurrence
		Cases	Joints			Pain	Swelling	Mobility	Deformity	
Wilde, Sawmiller	1969	23	69	PIP	30 months	35 joints (occas. intense) 26 9)	10 joints	ROM decrease 30–50°–3 joints. Mobility as preop. or improved.–others		
Kemesi	1971	37 (40 hands)	97	MCP	6–36 months	none 25 slight 12 intense 3		Active passive <80° 21% 44% 40–80° 54% 40% 40° 22% 10%	Function of hands: normal 18 subnorm. 18 decreased 4	
Ellison, Kelly, Flatt	1971	67	390	MCP PIP	3 months–10 years (av. 4.5 yrs.)	33 cases (but less than preop.)	20 cases	57 cases ROM decrease < 15°	38 cases	
Pahle	1973	93 (114 hands)	233	PIP	2 months–5 years (av. 26 months)	7 joints	none 48 slight 141 visible 44	flex. contracture av. 0–45° (11°) ROM 50–110 (87°)	7 joints	4 cases
Wilde	1974	34	98	PIP	1 year–5.8 years (av. 36.5 months)	none 73 decreased 14 as preoper. 11	30%	average decrease 4°		7 joints with swelling + pain

When we compare the reports of several authors who have published their synovectomy reports in recent years, we obtain the picture shown in Tables 1 and 2.

There is practically general agreement in most of the papers on synovectomy (knee and finger joints), that

A. Positive

1. It has a favourable effect on the pain and thus usually a positive influence on the function.

2. It enables us to eliminate or reduce the swelling

3. It has no appreciable influence on the mobility of the operated joint.

B. Negative

4. The result depends on the degree of preoperative destruction and therefore we find a relatively frequent deterioration of the X-ray picture after the operation.

5. There is a gradual deterioration in the clinical result as time goes on after the operation and so:

An increase of recurrent synovitis in the years following the operation is to be expected.

On the other hand, opinions are divided in how far synovectomy, particularly in the case of a larger joint, is able to influence the entire process, that is the activity of the disease and thus the progress on the other nonoperated joints.

Above all, however, there is a lack of comparable studies dealing with the progress of the disease on operated and non-operated joints, especially where comparable observations of the synovitic involvement of joints could be made. Apart from the ethical dubiousness and psychological difficulties, which must entail the holding back of an operation, which has been found successful on one side, from the opposite side, conclusions, according to unknown prognosis of every RA and the often capricious different course on the individual joints, for which we have no explanation, may only be drawn with care. When we analyse the criteria, according to which the majority of successes in respect of synovectomy are measured, one is astonished that the results do not differ to any greater extent and namely because of the following reasons:

1. *The non-uniformity of the groups of patients on which the statistics are based*
a) according to sex
b) according to age
c) according to profession. Depending on the physical strain on the operated joints, we must expect different results.
d) according to the duration of the disease
e) according to the number of affected joints
f) according to the immunological parameter
g) according to the stage of illness: a rough classification into early and late synovectomy is not fair particularly to the last group where some of the degrees of destruction vary to a considerable extent
h) according to the time after the operation. Although it would be possible to make a comparison of sufficiently large groups over analogous periods of time, only a few of the statistics known to us pursue one and the same case over periods of months and years.

i) according to the histological picture

k) according to disease activity at the time of the re-examination.

2. There is no consideration of the drug therapy applied prior to, during and after the operation. The type and effectiveness of the medications, in particular the analgetics, possibly even steroid applications, influence or falsify the operation results as well under certain conditions.

3. The different operation and after-treatment techniques of various surgeons not only influence the radical character of the synovectomy and thus perhaps the extent of the recurrence quota, but also – depending on the operative approach – the degree of traumatizing of the tissue, which influences the success of the operation in respect to post-operative pain, mobility and secondary osteoarthritis.

4. There is no uniform follow-up-examination (several examiners, assessment on the basis of the case history only).

5. Various criteria are used for the follow-up: Different interpretation of the rating "good". Different assessments of the swelling, quite often without any differentiation as to whether it concerns a soft tissue, a recurrent synovitis or a sensitive knee in the case of secondary osteoarthritis.

We shall consider the problems of defining a recurrent synovitis in more detail later.

6. The influence of synovectomy on the radiological aspect is also interpreted quite differently. Here, it is not only the well known difficulties, e.g. the impossibility of detecting localized lesion, even if severe in large joints, such as in knee joints (and the great differences in some cases depending on the projection) that play a role, but also the most astonishing and striking fact is that the evaluation of the X-rays was obviously effected without the use of a point-system and so it is left more or less to the subjective influence of the examiner, which is diastrous with a number of examiners.

The rating of the success with very good, good, satisfactory and poor, or their equivalent, is justified in such cases where a subjective assessment of the patients is desired. The objective measurement for the effectiveness of the synovectomy – as was applied in the mentioned statistics – is associated with a decisive disadvantage, namely that it tends to compare the post-operative state with the normal condition instead of considering individually the gain or loss in points in comparison with the pre-operative condition.

Concretely, this means that the complete elimination of pain in the case of a late synovectomy with marked swelling may be rated as a very good result if movement is still not normal but nevertheless better than it was post-operatively. This is not the case, however, with an early synovectomy which does not result in a normal range of motion or where occasional sweling occurs. The actual condition compared with the normal one is less decisive for the results assessment than the extent of the gain in points, which constitutes the degree of improvement or deterioration in comparison with the post-operative state.

3. Our synovectomy study

3.1 *Method*

In an endeavour to determine the value of synovectomy in a better manner and to complement the subjective components of the re-examination through as many objective and reproducible data as possible, we have proceeded as follows in the re-examination of 100 knee and 370 finger synovectomies.

3.1.1 The same person – a doctor with rheumatological training – who is more objective to the operation results than the operating surgeon conducted the examinations.

3.1.2 Examinations at regular intervals after 3, 6, 12 and 24 months and in some cases, 3, 4 and 5 years after the operation.

3.1.3 The examinations were made according to a so-called orthopaedic examination sheet, which considers primarily the morphological and functional side of the patient and a so-called rheumatological sheet that is purposed, above all, to the serological-humoral aspects of the illness.

3.1.4 Regular X-ray checks were made on the operated and non-operated knee joints in the case of knee synovectomy patients and both hands ap for the synovectomy of finger joints. The simple ap pictures were supplemented by *Norgard's* ball-catching and *Brewerton's* special projection-X-ray. The assessment and comparison of the pre- and post-operative pictures was made by the same doctor. His verdict was then compared with that of a second doctor, who worked independently.

3.1.5 Since the same surgeon performed the operation in over 80% of all the knee- and in more than 90% of all the finger-synovectomies, there was no significant difference in respect to the operating technique and after-treatment.

3.1.6 The mentioned examination comprises a total check up of the locomotor system and therefore allows the fate of non-operated joints and tendon sheets to be followed exactly as well, and – as a result of several functional tests – examination of the extent of invalidity. Furthermore, by way of a large number of serological reports, it is possible to determine the activity at the time of the respective re-examination and in a regular time sequence. The medication rendered earlier and at the time of the examination is recorded accurately on the same sheet.

3.1.7 In the case of knee synovectomy the synovial fluid is examined in relation to immunological and enzymatical parameter.

3.1.8 The synovectomy specimens were examined by two pathologists specially trained in this field.

3.1.9 In 10 cases of knee synovectomy, where the re-examination revealed swelling of the joint with effusion and the decision of whether a recurrent synovitis was present appeared impossible (see below), we examined the punctate concerning the serological parameter for RA (verification of rheumatic factor, immune complex and enzyme activity) – ad 3.1.3 Examination System.

Fig. 1 shows the orthopaedic and rheumatological examination sheets (see *Winer, Böni*).

Tab. 3 represents the 18-point system employed for the evaluation of the X-ray of the knee joint.

Tab. 4 the 18-point system for the finger joint X-rays.

The evaluation is effected according to a point system which, in our opinion, has an advantage over the group classification, namely that it is less exposed to the subjectivity of the assessment. Furthermore, the point ratings facilitate graphical re-presentation of the treatment successes as a function of the time that has passed since the operation.

The following parameter are determined point-wise for the knee and the operated finger joints: Pain, swelling, mobility, deformity and X-ray picture. In accordance with the peculiarities of the knee and finger joints, the parameter points may be defined as follows (see also Tab. 5 & 6).

Knee joint (Tab. 5)

In the case of pain, swelling, mobility and deformity, the normal condition is shown as zero. The mode of classification facilitates improved graphical representation of the pathological deviation in the coordinate system. Three points are given as the poorest rating for each parameter. Consequently four ratings are possible for each parameter, namely 0, 1, 2 and 3. Since deformities include a number of components, the points score has been sub-divided. The lack of extension has been given a rating analogous with a varus or valgus deformity combined with instability, that is collateral ligament insufficiency of the joint. In other words, we rate an extension lack of more than 30° the same as a varus deformity of more than 20°, accompanied with an instability of more than 20° side movement.

Finger joints (Tab. 6)

With the finger joints, conditions were more complicated because here specific deformities occur (ulnar/radial deviation, boutonnière or swanneck deformity), which tend to influence the functional result to a significant degree. The rating classification has been made in keeping with *Swanson* et al. (see Fig. 1). The code numbers for the respective parameters are shown in parentheses. "Deformity" and "Instability", which were summarized under a single parameter for the knee joints, had to be defined individually.

Table 3. X-ray evaluation of the knee joint after synovectomy.
(Evaluate each joint separately.)

Last name:	First name:		Age:		
No. of case history _____	Joint: _____		R / L		
Date: _____	pre-op.		post-op.		
	months	months	months	months	months

Articular space normal	0					
narrowed by $^1/_3$	1					
narrowed by $^2/_3$	2					
narrowed by more than $^2/_3$	3					
Articular space relatively same	0					
up to $^1/_2$ narrower	1					
more than $^1/_2$ narrower	2					
deformation med. = X						
deformation lat. = O						
Erosion and cysts						
none	0					
single small	1					
single large or many small	2					
Irregular contours of articular space						
none	0					
slight irregularity	0					
very irregular, wavy or break	2					
Secondary osteoarthritic changes						
none	0					
i.e. osteophytes,						
single, small	1					
several, small/medium	2					
massiv osteophythosis	3					
Sclerosis						
none	0					
slightly increased	1					
massiv with rubble-cysts	2					
Osteoporosis						
none	0					
slight	1					
marked	2					
Subluxation						
none	0					
slight	1					
severe	2					
Total points		/6	/6	/6	/6	/6

Final score   1/6 — 6/6 = 1
(0—1—2—3)   7/6 — 12/6 = 2
            13/6 — 18/6 = 3

Comments:
Development of polyarthritic changes:
Development of osteoarthritic changes:

        deterioration
        severe deterioration
        same
        improvement

Operative findings:
(Especially clarification of the question to what extent the operative findings correspond with the X-ray evaluation before surgery.)

                                                     Name of evaluator

with the fingers because they frequently occur independently of each other. This is why we have laid down 5 parameter with a maximum points score of 15 here instead of 4 with a total score of 12. With the finger joints, pain and swelling are rated in the same way as for knee joints.

The X-rays of synovectomized joints were evaluated individually (according to the partly very different degrees of destruction of the various finger joints of one hand). With the aid of an 18-point system, we have endeavoured to summarize all the possible signs of destruction, particularly the specifically polyarthritic ones, according to their significance, and to differentiate same from secondary osteoarthritic changes. A total points score of 18 was selected because it could be divided by a factor of 6, i.e. a figure equal to the clinical parameter and could be included with this in an overall rating.

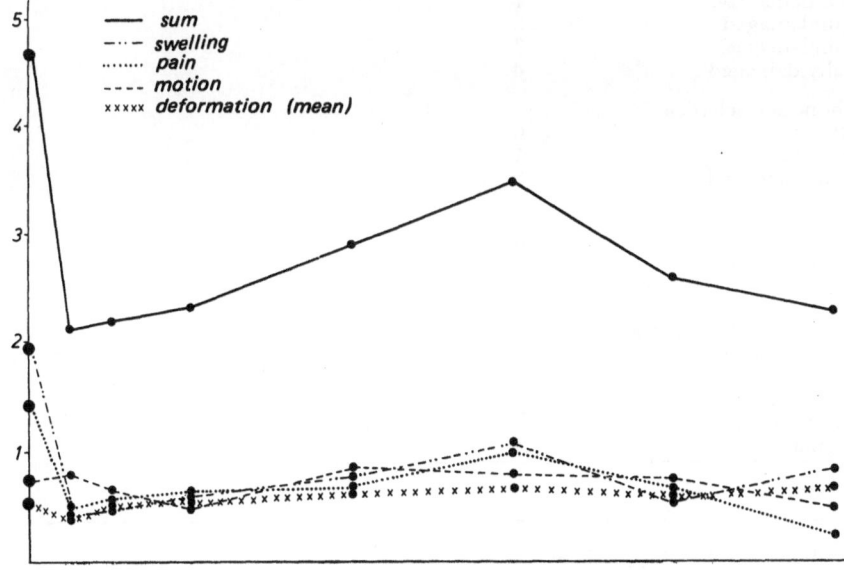

Fig. 2. Knee synovectomy-results (100) over a period of 5 years.

Table 4

Evaluation of x-ray of the finger joints after synovectomy

	MCP	PIP	DIP
a	1	1	1
b	2	2	2
c	3	3	3
d	4	4	4
e	5	5	5

(For each joint evaluate separately)

Last name: First name: Age: | right / left |

Case history no.:

Date:

	preoperative	postoperative	
	months	months	months

Articular space
 normal   0
 narrowed to ½   1
 narrowed by more than ½   2

Erosions and cysts
 none   0
 disturbed trabecula structur   1
 single small cysts in otherwise
 undamaged joints   2
 separate large cysts in otherwise
 undamaged joints   3
 many small cysts   4
 many large cysts   5

Joint surface
 undamaged   0
 ²/₃ undamaged   1
 ½ undamaged   2
 ⅓ undamaged   3
 totally damaged   4

Subchondrale sclerosis
 constant   0
 interrupted   1
 totally damaged   2

Osteoporosis
 none   0
 in proximity of joint   1
 diffuse   2

Subluxation and dislocation,
loss of surface contact
 none   0
 less than 50%   1
 more than 50%   2
 complete   3

Total points   /6

End results   1/6 — 6/6 = 1
(0—1—2—3)   7/6 — 12/6 = 2
                    13/6 — 18/6 = 3

Table 5. Definition of parameter for the evaluation of the results of knee synovectomie

Evaluation principles of local operative results

Pain	Swelling	Mobility (flexion)
0 — none	0 — none	0 — 125° or more
1 — occasional	1 — visible	1 — 110—125°
2 — on weight-bearing	2 — distinct	2 — 90—110°
3 — at rest	3 — > 10%	3 — < 90°

Loss of extension	Instability	Varus deformity	Valgus deformity
0 — complete	0 — none	0 — none	0 — none
½ — 5 — 10°	¼ — to 10°	¼ — to 10°	¼ — to 20°
1 — 10 — 30°	½ — to 20°	½ — 10 — 20°	½ — 20 — 30°
1½ — > 30°	¾ — > 20°	¾ — > 20°	¾ — > 45°

Table 6. Definition of parameter for the evaluation of the results of finger synovectomies

I Pain

    0 — none
    1 — occasional
    2 — on weight-bearing
    3 — at rest

II Swelling

    0 — none
    1 — visible
    2 — distinct
    3 — 10%

III Range of motion (ROM)

MCP, DIP, IP	PIP	Thumb MCP
0 — 70° or more	0 — 90° or more	0 — 40° or more
1 — 50° to 70°	1 — 70° to 90°	1 — 30° to 40°
2 — 30° to 50°	2 — 50° to 70°	2 — 20° to 30°
3 — less than 30°	3 — less than 50°	3 — less than 20°

IV Deformity

MCP fingers Ulnar or radial drift	MCP thumb boutonnière	MCP fingers swan-neck	boutonnière
0 — none			
1 — 0° to 10°	1 — −5° to −20°	1 — +10° to 50°	1 — −5° to −10°
2 — 10° to 30°	2 — −20° to −40°	2 — +20° to 30°	2 — −10° to −30°
3 — more than 30°	3 — more than −40°	3 — +30° to 10°	3 — more than −30°

V Instability

Instability	Subluxation
0 — none	0 — none
½ — 0° to 10°	½ — mild
1 — 10° to 20°	1 — moderate
1½ — more than 20°	1½ — severe

3.2 *Casuistry*

72 patients with 100 knee synovectomies and 80 patients with 370 finger synovectomies were analysed.

The sex, age, duration of illness, stage of illness and number of simultaneously affected joints in the case of patients with knee synovectomies, are shown in Tables 7–11.

As expected, these tables reveal a high predominance of female patients (80% of all patients). A further typical observation is that more than 80% of all the patients are aged between 20 and 60, with the peak between 40 and 45. The somewhat surprising observation that the disease was already in an advanced stage in the case of approximately 75% of all the patients, i.e. *Steinbrocker* stage 3–4, is definitely of significance for correct assessment of the results. This is also confirmed by the fact that the duration of illness prior to the operation in the case of more than 50% of the patients was over 10 years, whereas only 10% of those who underwent an operation had been ill for less than 2 years.

In other words, we only performed an early synovectomy in exceptional cases, the majority of patients had late synovectomies.

Further information is provided on the serological analysis of the patients and the question of pre-operative medical treatment in the rheumatological section.

Table 7. Knee synovectomy

n = 72	
Male	19%
Female	81%

Table 8. Age of patient before knee synovectomy

n = 72	
under 20 years	9,8%
21–40 years	37,3%
41–60 years	43,1%
over 60 years	9,8%

Table 9. Duration of the illness before synovectomy

n = 72	
less than 2 years	10,4%
2–5 years	18,2%
6–10 years	15,4%
more than 10 years	56,0%

Table 10. Stage of illness according to Steinbrocker before knee synovectomy

n = 72	
Stage of illness I	9,7%
Stage of illness II	20,8%
Stage of illness III	47,2%
Stage of Illness IV	22,3%

Table 11. Synovectomy and type of affected joints

monoarticular	2%
oligoarticular*)	13%
polyarticular	85%
*) oligoarticular = up to 5 small joints	
or 1–3 large joints	

3.3 *Results from the orthopaedic standpoint*

3.3.1 When we speak here from the orthopaedic standpoint, we mean the criteria pain, swelling, mobility, deformity and X-rays that were recorded as a part of our survey and which are of particular interest to operating orthopaedic surgeons. The graphs (Tab. 2 & 3) show all the added parameter in the upper summation curve. The behaviour during the course of the post-operative period is clearly visible. Below this curve are those showing the individual parameter for pain, swelling, mobility and deformity. The summation curve begins at a high level because most were late synovectomies drops during the first 3 and 6 months and then rises again.

Nevertheless, it still does not rise to the level at the outset, that means on average, the result – three years after the operation – is still always better than prior to the operation. In addition, it is noticeable that the condition does not necessarily deteriorate in the fourth and fifth post-operative year, in fact it improves somewhat. Nevertheless, it should be considered that only a part of all the operated joints (25 knee, 45 finger) are included in the five-year statistics. The parameter curves for pain and swelling drop remarkably in the first 1/2 year. Noticeable is the more or less conformity of the knee and finger synovectomies. When we compare the summation curve with those for the individual parameter, we also find that the rise or the deterioration in the results two and three years after the operation is attributable in the majority of cases to an increase of the deformity. On the other hand, the symptoms that represented the main indication for an operation, i.e. pain and swelling, continue to run in a considerably more favourable deeper area. The increase in deformity is not at all surprising because

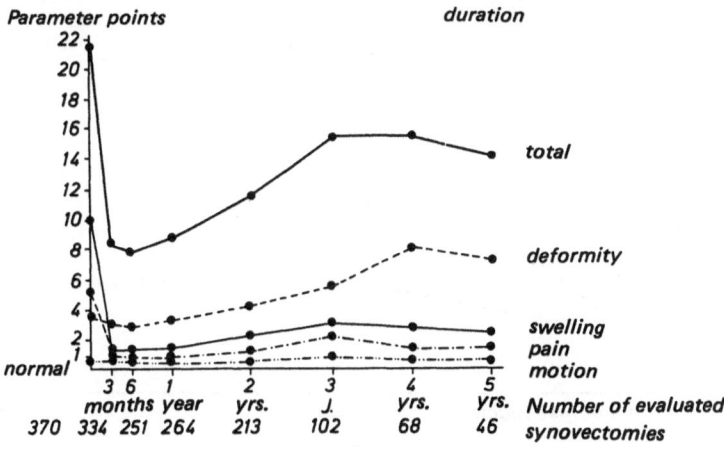

Fig. 3. Finger synovectomy-results

most of cases are late synovectomies. This development becomes very clear when we follow the X-ray parameter curve which shows – as is to be expected – a deterioration in the case of late synovectomy. The different clinical behaviour of early and late synovectomy could also be observed through the separate representation of the parameter summation curves for cases of early and late synovectomy. In this case, the level of the start ng value determines the end figure or, in other words, the lower the parameter value at the outset, respectively the degree of joint damage at the time of the operation, the lower, the end value will be. With actual early synovectomies (stage 1), an improvement is even found over the entire observation period, and leads to a more or less normal condition. The favourable course of the synovectomy in respect to mono- and oligoarticular cases can be seen on Tab. 5.

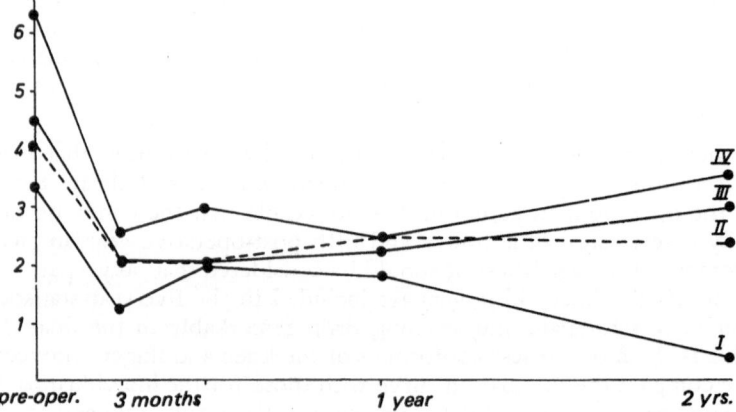

Fig. 4. Knee synovetomy-results. Postoperative time elapse according to stage of illness

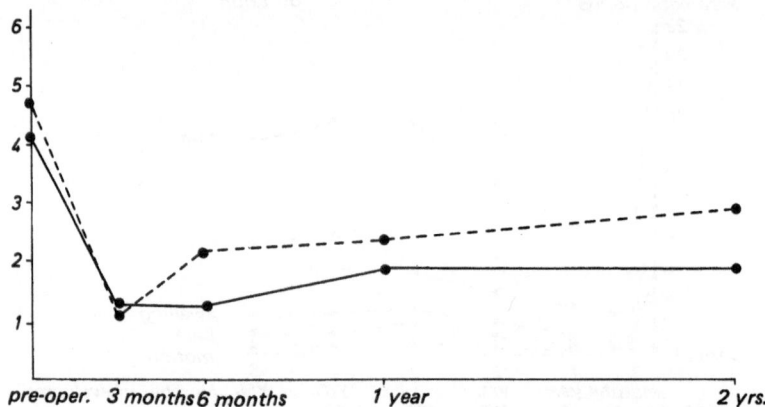

Fig. 5. Knee synovectomy-results — — — oligo- and monoarticular cases,
— — — Total average

Although the parameter curves reflect the behaviour of the individual symptoms over the course of the post-operative period quite clearly, Figures 6–11 provide quantitatively better information on the percentual ratio of improved/unchanged and deteriorated cases. In the finger synovectomies, the clinical overall assessment and an analysis of the five-year results are plotted for the individual parameter (Fig. 8–11). (The number of operated joints decreases as the period after the operation increases.) Here again the predominantly positive influence of the synovectomy on pain and swelling becomes evident, whereas mobility does not undergo any striking change.

Cases, which were free of pain pre-operatively and where persistent swelling gave indication to the necessity of an operation, were painful for a time under certain conditions post-operatively, and then became free of pain in the majority of cases.

3.3.2 The *analysis of the X-rays* of the knee joint (see Fig. 12–14 and Tab.) prior to and after the operation were accorded particular care, because they were purposed to providing conclusive evidence as to the expected final result, respectfully the eventual necessity of a subsequent reconstructive operation. Whereas with finger joint destructional changes in the subchondral bone are relatively easy to determine – due to the smaller dimensions – particularly when in addition to the customary ap views, the ball catching and special X-ray of *Norgard* and *Brewerton* are employed – difficulties of a much greater extent are encountered with knee joints. Firstly, because the lesions in many cases of synovectomy – and not only with the pronounced early synovectomies – are often strongly localized and only concern the cartilage. How should one detect a thick pannus and the subjacent severe cartilage damage from the X-ray, or an erosion extending to the bone, which lies in the middle of an otherwise fully normal joint surface and thus does not reduce the joint space.Even large erosions in the center of the joint surface may not be seen when surrounded by healthy cartilage on either side. On the other hand, positioning of the knee joint is of great importance. Thus the elimination or the occurrence of an extension deficit in the knee joint will also influence the width of the interarticular space not allowing us to draw conclusions as to an improvement or deterioration of the joint surface. Cysts, pseudocysts and erosions are usually only recognizable in an X-ray when they have minimum dia-

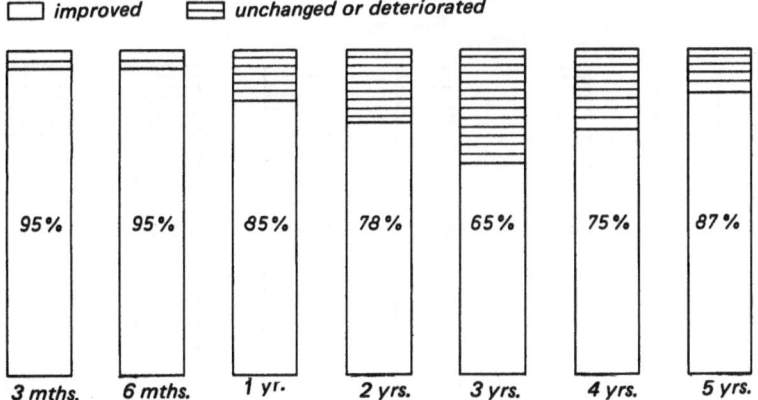

Fig. 6. Knee synovectomies during a period of 5 years

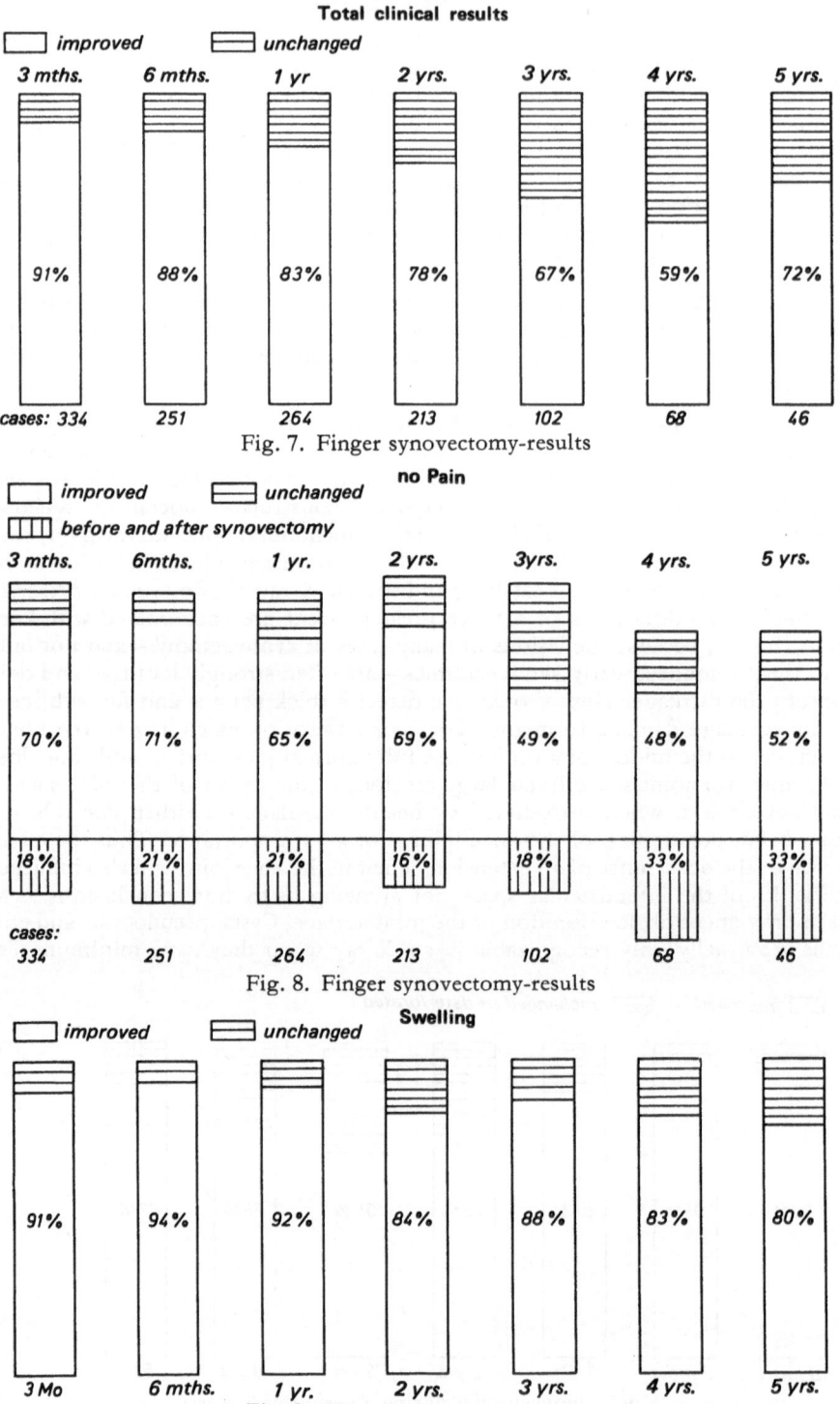

Total clinical results

☐ improved   ⊟ unchanged

| 3 mths. | 6 mths. | 1 yr | 2 yrs. | 3 yrs. | 4 yrs. | 5 yrs. |

91% 88% 83% 78% 67% 59% 72%

cases: 334   251   264   213   102   68   46

Fig. 7. Finger synovectomy-results

no Pain

☐ improved   ⊟ unchanged

▥ before and after synovectomy

| 3 mths. | 6mths. | 1 yr. | 2 yrs. | 3yrs. | 4 yrs. | 5 yrs. |

70% 71% 65% 69% 49% 48% 52%

18% 21% 21% 16% 18% 33% 33%

cases:
334   251   264   213   102   68   46

Fig. 8. Finger synovectomy-results

Swelling

☐ improved   ⊟ unchanged

91% 94% 92% 84% 88% 83% 80%

| 3 Mo | 6 mths. | 1 yr. | 2 yrs. | 3 yrs. | 4 yrs. | 5 yrs. |

Fig. 9. Finger synovectomy-results

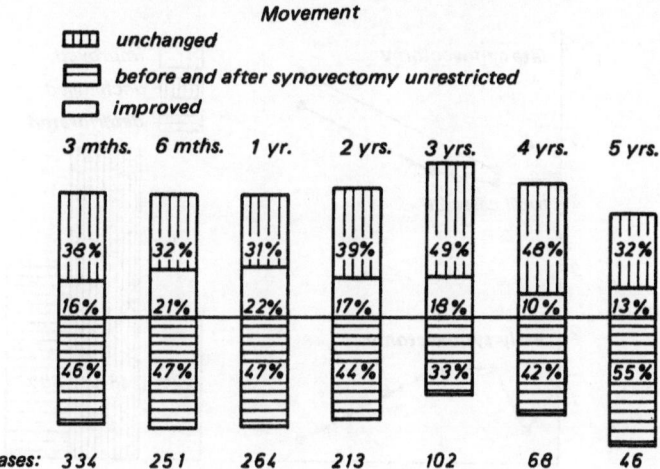

Fig. 10. Finger synovectomy-results

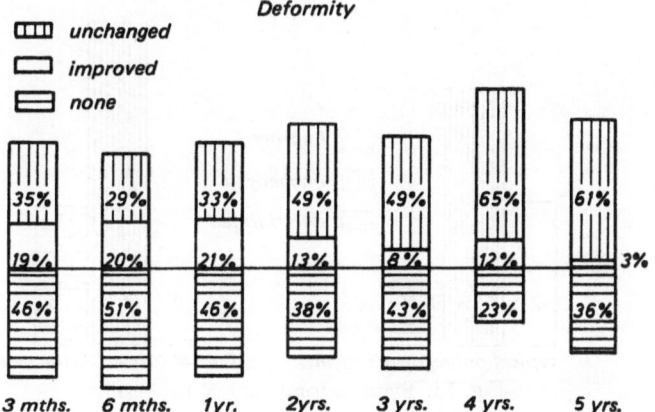

Fig. 11. Finger synovectomy-results

meters of 1 to 1,5 cm; numerous small defects, which are not any more favourable prognostically, may not be seen. We must be careful not to interpret physiological indentations of the bone as erosions, especially when these occur quite suddenly in a follow-up series during slight rotation of the knee joint. Joint gap widening however, can also simulate an improvement in the case of partial joint collapse as long as we do not take X-rays under load. For comparison with X-rays made earlier, we must then call for the same projection. The assessment of the behaviour of osteoporosis is also difficult or even impossible, whereas secondary osteo-arthritic changes are somewhat easier to appreciate. It is important to look out for fine irregularities in the joint space.

The evaluation of the X-rays is plotted in Figures 12–14. Of 86 knee synovectomies, we were able to examine the series of X-rays prior to and at regular intervals after the operation. It was established that,

1. generally speaking, the X-ray picture changed very little,

2. an analysis of the individual cases showed an improvement in 22% and a deterioration in 30% of the cases.

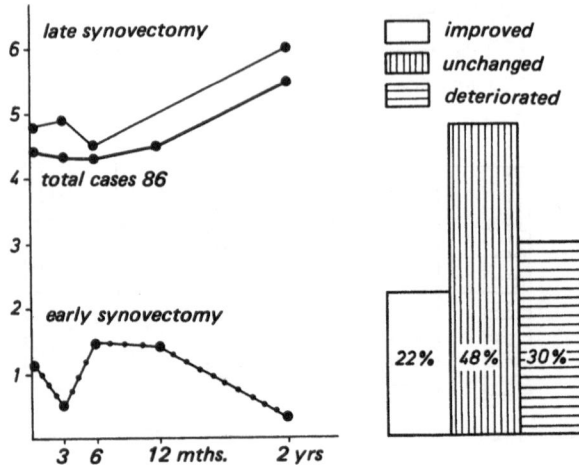

Fig. 12. Synovectomy and X-ray results

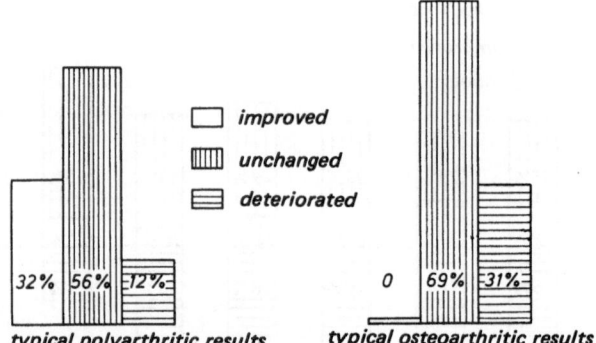

Fig. 13. Synovectomy and X-ray results

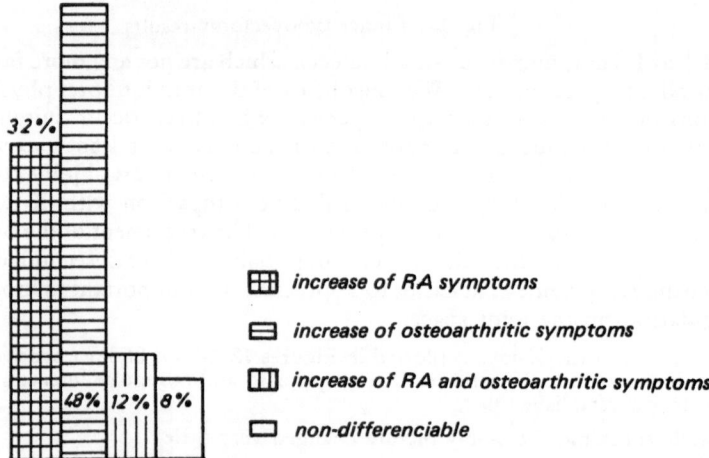

Fig. 14. Knee synovectomy and X-ray finding differentiation of the deterioration

3. When we consider the group where an improvement in the X-ray picture is confirmed, we find in the majority of cases that there has been a retrogression of the typical polyarthritic changes (osteoporosis, erosions).

4. On the other hand, the group where the X-ray picture shows a deterioration, it is established that the deterioration is associated with

48% typical osteoarthritic changes
32% typical polyarthritic symptoms
12% combination of both, and in
 2% no safe assessment was possible.

5. Behaviour analysis of the radiological typical polyarthritic changes for the complete serie resulted in

an improvement in 32% of the cases
a deterioration in 12%, and
no change in 56%.

Figure 15 and Fig. 16 provide an examples of where there was an improvement in the polyarthritic changes.

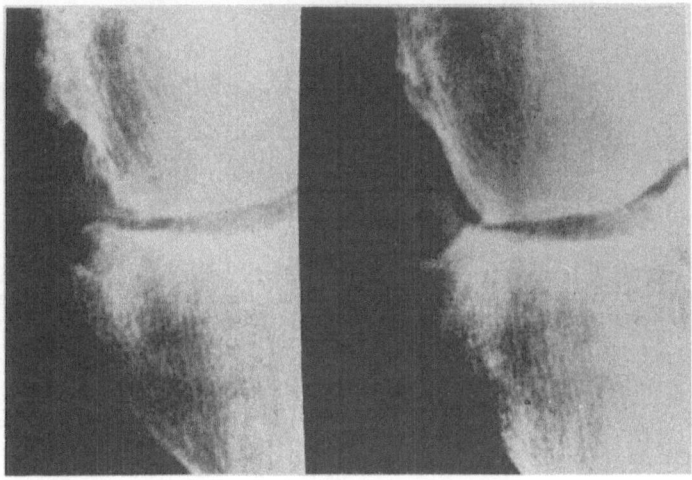

Fig. 15. Left knee before synovectomy; right knee after synovectomy. The joint contours are smooth, the marginal erosion seems to be partially filled, a finding which also other authors (*Ansell*) could prove.

6. Behaviour analysis of the radiological typical osteoarthritic changes in the complete series showed

an improvement in 0% of the cases
a deterioration in 31%, and
no change in 60%.

7. When we make a special consideration of the behaviour of the X-rays in the case of early synovectomies (12%) and late synovectomies (88%), we can observe the following behaviour:

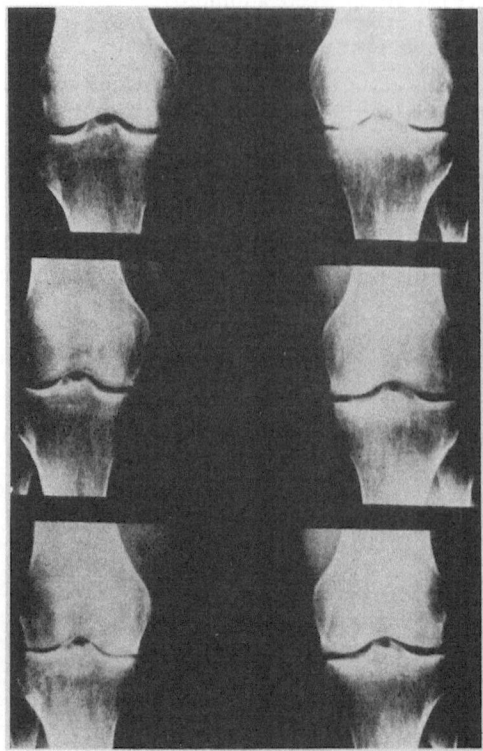

Fig. 16. A series of X-rays taken over a period of many years of the non-operated knee joint (left) and the synovectomized knee joint (right). The deterioration of the initially improved and therefore non-operated knee joint is just as evident as the improvement of the synovectomized right knee.

	early synovectomies	late synovectomies
improvement	20%	22%
deterioration	20%	31%
no change	60%	47%

As is expected, the X-ray picture deteriorates more frequently with late than early synovectomies.

8. With the early synovectomies, the improvements are exclusively improvements in the polyarthritic changes, and the deteriorations exclusively deteriorations in the osteo-arthritic changes.

9. The X-rays of the 22 patients which showed no clinical improvement during re-examination (no change or worse than pre-operatively) were subject to a special analysis. It was found that there was a deterioration in the X-ray picture in 41% (30%), improvement 14% (22%) and no change in 45% (48%) of the cases. The figures in parentheses are analogue values for the total collection of 86 knee joints.

From this, it follows that the clinical deterioration in general is only visible to a slight extent in the X-ray picture.

10. Of 76 late synovectomies (cases where at operation destruction on the cartilage was confirmed), 11 had roentgenologically inconspicuous joints (no narrowing of the interarticular space, no erosions) = 14%.

Table 12. Late results of knee synovectomy

Number of patients	77
Sex: ♀ 63 ♂ 14	
Number of operated knees	100
(in 23 patients both knees)	
Side: R 54 L 46	
Time after operation	
minimum	4 years
maximum	11 years
average	6,2 years

Table 13. Late results of knee synovectomy

Pain		Number of knees
None		42
Occassional	in motion/under load 38	40
	at rest 9	
Constant	in motion/under load 18	18
	at rest 7	

Table 14. Late results of knee synovectomy

Swelling		Number of knees
None		45
Slight	occassional 29	34
	constant 5	
Medium	occassional 10	16
	constant 6	
Severe		5

Table 15. Late results of knee synovectomy

Punctures in past year	Number of knees
once	8
more often	15

Table 16. Late results of knee synovectomy

Walking ability		Number of patients
Unlimited		42
Limited to	100 m 2	34
	500 m 11	
	1 km 21	
Unable to walk		1

Table 17. Late results of knee synovectomy

Reason for restricted ability to walk	Number
Operated knee	33
Another knee	9
Hip	19
	26

Table 18. Late results of knee synovectomy

Motion			
Flexion	Number of knees	Extension	Number of knees
over 90°	68	full	68
up tp 90°	22	up to 20°	30
up to 60°	10	over 20°	2

Table 19. Late results of knee synovectomy

Climbing stairs		Number of patients
without aid		53
with cane/canes		12
only with banister	possible	9
	impossible	3

Table 20. Late results of knee synovectomy

Walking aid	Number of patients
without	55
with	22

Table 21. Late results of knee synovectomy

Deformity			Number of knees
None			63
Varus	slight	13	13
	severe	0	
Valgus	slight	12	21
	severe	9	
Flail joint	slight	12	20
	severe	8	

3.3.3 **Analysis of the X-ray pictures for finger synovectomies.** Statistically, the deterioration in the analysis of 300 finger joint synovectomies concerned 149 cases, i.e. 50%, if we consider a point difference of 1 as a deterioration. Proceeding from the assumption that with an 18-points score system the difference of 1 point could still lie within the error limit, we determined the cases which exhibited a post-operative points increase of at least 3 points, i.e. a definite deterioration. This was established in 57 cases or 19% of all the examined joints.

If we wish to assess the value of synovectomy on the basis of the X-ray, we are apt to compare the spontaneous development of a non-operated side (finger or knee joints) with the operated side when clinical changes occur symmetrically. The differing destruction of the individual joints, which can manifest itself on the various joints of one hand, must be considered as well when comparing the analogous jonts of both hands, just like the different loadings (extra loading of the joint of the right hand in the case of a right-handed person), simulatneous medications etc.

In considering all these factors, it can be clearly established through the analysis of the series of X-rays that destruction is prevented or at least delayed for a time by the synovectomy.

Nowadays, when greater interest is shown in chemical and radioisotopic synovectomy (see below), we feel that clarification as to the effective duration of operative synovectomy is of paramount importance. As already stated, the number of cases with an observation period of more than 3 years was relatively small in the analysis which we completed more than 3 years ago, the results of which are shown in Figure 6. As the outcome of these cases must be of interest to us, we re-examined 77 patients with 100 operated knee joints. The re-examination involved 63 women and 14 men. The period since the operation was minimum 4, maximum 11 and on average 6,2 years. The results are shown in Tables 12–22.

Table 22. Late Results of knee synovectomy—evaluation

Pain	Swelling	Walking ability	Mobility	Classification		Comparison of condition pre- and post-operatively	Point score	Number of knees	Results
				Deformities	Instability				
None	None, occassional or slight	Unlimited	Flex. 110° > ext. full	None	None	Improvement	0–3	42	Considerable Improvement
Occassional	Distinct, occasional	Limited up to 1 km	Flex. 90–110° ext. full	Slight	Slight	Improvement	4–6	30	Improvement
Constant	Severe and constant	Considerably restricted or unable to walk	Flex < 90° loss of extension	Severe	Severe	Unchanged or deteriorated	over 6	28	Deterioration

They show that in more than one third of the cases, the operated knee joint does not exhibit any pain or swelling. More than 50% of the patients could walk without restriction. Mobility was especially good, because it exceeded 90° in more than two thirds of the re-examined patients. Here again, we must not forget the large number of late synovectomies (81%) among the patients. Including the knee joints, where pain and swelling only occurred occasionally and to a slight degree, the proportion of patients for which such an operation was worthwhile, is more than 3/4 of all the cases under review. When we again consider the high number of late synovectomies by which, apart from the synovectomy – further operations were necessary (with the knee, for example meniscectomy and removal of softened and worn parts of the cartilage: with the finger joints recentering and reefing of the extensor mechanism), the operative synovedtomy may be regarded as definitely superior to chemical and radioisotope synovectomy in stages 2 and 3. We also agree with other authors *(Vainio, Laine* and *Vainio, Jakubowski, Brattström)* that chemical and radioisotope synovectomy has its domain in the early stages of synovitis and anyone performing it must be prepared to repeat the operative synovectomy in case of failure.

The predominantly positive influence of synovectomy on the operated joint is clearly shown by the hitherto graphical analysis. However, opinions differ as to the influence on the general disease activity of other localizations. Whereas an attempt is made to answer this question in the rheumatological part of this publication by analysing the influence of synovectomy on the laboratory tests, we compared the degree of invalidity among synovectomized patients prior to and after the operation at the time of various re-examinations (according to the *Steinbrocker* grades). The curves in Tab. 17 show quite clearly that, despite improvement in the condition at the operated joint (summation curve of the parameter), the disability continues to progress slowly. In this particular case, it should be remembered again that the majority of these patients were late synovectomies and had been sick for more than 10 years in 56% of the cases and with a polyarthritic activity in 85%.

3.4 *Recurrent synovitis*

The question of *recurrent synovitis* has never been answered satisfactorily, particularly as to the frequency of its occurrence is concerned.

There is no general agreement on the definition of recurrent synovitis and, which and how many histological criteria are required in light microscopy for the diagnosis of a recurrent synovitis. To which of these criteria and to what extent should a specific character be approved? On the other hand, statements have been made by *Hirohata* and *Morimoto*, that in the ultra microscopy the regenerated synovium is qualitatively very similar to the removed diseased synovium and that there are only quantitative differences in the majority of cases.

In view of the fact that the majority of synovectomies are late ones, recurrent swellings can frequently be explained by reduced stability, chondromalacia, etc. So we can only progress further through routine biopsy. Shall we subject patients, which occasionally do not suffer from the recurring swelling, to a further operation?

The problem of recurrent synovitis is to be discussed later.

4. Chemical and Radioisotope-synovectomy

To an increasing degree and in selected cases, *Chemical and Radioisotope-synovectomy* (wynoviorthesis) constitutes an effective alternative to operative synovectomy. Since on the one hand, there were only few references to the subject in the German language and on the other, the discussion of results with operative synovectomy call for knowledge of the possibilities with synoviorthesis, we shall deal with this procedure in more detail.

When we consider the temporal and financial efforts involved, the physical and psychological stress placed on the patient with every operation or even a number of operations, as is frequently the case with RA, not to mention the possibility of complications and the uncertainty of the long-term result, we can well understand the efforts that have been made for a long time to eliminate the diseased synovium through intra-articular injection of certain obliterating substances or radioisotopes.

Whereas the first tests with chemical synovectomy and osmic acid can be traced back to *V. Reis* and *Swensson* (1951), radioactive colloids were used by *Ansell, Crook, Mallard* and *Bywaters* in 1963, by *Makin* and *Robin* in 1964. The following agents have been used for chemical synovectomy:

Thiotepa *(Flatt 1962, Fearnley 1964, Zuckner et al. 1966, Mondragon Kalb 1965 and Gross 1963)*

Osmic acid *(Reis 1951, Berglöf 1964, Martio 1972, Menkes 1973, Brattström 1973, Jakubowski, Oka 1970)*

Varicocid *(Tillmann 1973)*

Gold *(Delbarre 1973)*

None of these agents had a real selective effect only on the synovial layer. Frequently all the articular structures were more or less affected. This was reflected in a considerably painful reaction, which induced a number of authors *(Jakubowski, Laine* and *Vainio, Brattström* et al.*)* to inject cortisone and a local anaesthetic at the same time. On the other hand, when using osmic acid, for example, the cartilage underwent a massive brown colouration, which allows a certain amount of scepticism to be held in respect of the assurances that no actual damage to the cartilage has been proven *(Reis* and *Swensson, Oka, Martio, Fellinger* and *Thumb)*. A further interesting factor is the findings of *Piattier-Piketty* et al. during tests with rabbits, namely that cartilage damage is much more dependent on the age of the rabbit than the dosage of the osmic acid.

The success statistics of the mentioned authors differ to a considerable extent. With *Thiotepa (Flatt, Fearnly, Zuckner* et al., *Mondragon Kalb, Gross)*, the short duration of the positive results (6–9 months) and their rather small number (25% according to *Gross*) are particularly noticeable.

With osmic acid, we find larger discrepancies, namely an unusually high success quota of 90–95% *(Boussina* and *Fallet)*, which is opposed by an improvement in only about 50% one year after treatment in other reports *(Martio, Menkes, Oka)*.

In the case of Varicocid *(Tillmann, Niculescu)*, the numbers are too small to prove any superiority of this method over the others (80% improvement with an observation period of 1 to 27 months). This same applies to the intra-articular gold injections employed according to *Delbarre, Lewis* and *Ziff* with success.

Added attention should be given, however, to the *Radioisotope synoviorthesis* with which, apart from the English *(Ansell* et al., *Gumpel* et al.*)* particularly the French *(Delbarre, Menkes* et al.*)* and the Scandinavan authors *(Oka, Virkunen)* have been able to gather positive experience.

The following *radioactive substances* are available: 198 Au, 90 Y citrate, 90 Y resin, Rhenium 186, Erbium 169, 90 Y Ferric hydroxide, Radium 224. A common feature associated with them is the application of locally effective β-rays on the absence of α-rays, which only have a superficial effect, but release substantially more energy and have a poor dosable, too brutal effect.

The *indication* for the application of the various radioisotopes depends on the γ-ray content, which unfortunately do not have their effect at the point of injection but at a further distance and according to the various penetration depths. Accordingly, the particularly deep-penetrating Yttrium 90 is selected as the substance for knee and hip joints, admittedly only for patients of over fifty years of age *(Delbarre, Oka, Gumpel, Kalliomäki)*. For younger patients, Osmic acid *(Menkes* 1973, *Matio* 1972, *Oka* 1974*)* is preferred. For finger and interphalangeal joints, the use of Erbium is recommended by *Delbarre, Menkes* et al (1973) for analogous reasons. Compared with Au 198, more and more interest has been shown recently in Rhenium 186 because of the reduced radiation and the more favourable effect, particularly in the case of medium-size joints (elbows, wrists, etc.) *(Delbarre, Meukes* et al.).

The injection techniques are described in more detail in the mentioned references. Apart from exact adherence to the dosage, the secure interarticular position of the needle (image amplifier control) is important, as well as the simultaneous injection of a local anaesthetic with steroid additive. The last measure helps to reduce the pain considerably. Immobilisation for at least forty-eight hours helps to prevent a more important migration of the substance to the distant parts of the body *(de la Chapelle* 1972, *Oka* 1970, *Memkes* 1973, *Roberts* 1973*)*.

Generally speaking, the results obtained with radioisotope-synoviorthesis appear to be superior to those attained with chemical synovectomy *(Delbarre* and *Menkes, Oka)*. An improvement was still observed in 80% of the cases even two years after the synoviorthesis. In 40%, very good results were estabilshed five years later. Another interesting factor is the dependency on the stage of the disease (clearly better results in the early stage) and the treated joint (more favourable results with knee joint than wrist joint). Yttrium 90 also appears to be definitely superior to Au 198 *(Oka* et al.*)*, particularly as well because with gold more than 10% of the injected quantity can migrate into the proximal lymph nodes *(Virkunen* 1967). More favourable reports on Au 198, however, have been given by *Fellinger* and *Thumb, Bauer, Gumpel* and *Stevenson*.

When we compare the results of chemical and radioisotope synovectomy with those of operative synovectomy, the former should be considered perhaps more frequently with the early synovectomy of joints, of course under due observation of the aforementioned measures.

The clear advantages of synoviorthesis are found in the
1. Simple technique
2. Reduced period of time in hospital
3. No narcotics

4. Low costs

5. Simple mobilization, and

6. Operative synovectomy still possible in the event of failure.

On the other hand, we should not forget the decisive disadvantages of synoviorthesis in comparison with operative synovectomy:

1. No application possibility in the case of tenosynovitis

2. Limited effect with multi-loculated joints (e. g. wrist joints) and with pronounced hypertropic villous synovitis

3. No reconstructive possibilities

4. Side effects (migration) which have not been completely clarified so far.

Although it is too early to establish definite boundaries between synoviorthesis and operative synovectomy, the indication for the application of Radioisotope synovectomy may be outlined as follows:

Early cases of mono- or oligoarticular synovitis without evidence (increasing importance of arthroscopy) for the presence of a severe hypertropic, villous synovitis in the case of seropositive and negative polyarthritis, as well as for

− Psoriasisarthritis

− Reiter syndrome

− Non-specific arthritis

− Villonodular synovitis

− Degenerative arthropathies with large effusions

− Hemophilia, and

− Ankylosing spondylitis.

The superiority of operative synovectomy remains undisputed in the case of tenosynovectomy and for late synovectomies of joints, where with the removal of the synovium reconstructive measures are necessary (recentering of the extensor mechanism on the finders, abrasion of the softened patellar cartilage, resection of a torn cartilage, suturing of overstretched ligaments in the knee, etc. Furthermore, with multi-loculated joints (wrist joint), where not all the joint sections can be reached by the injected substance, and with severe fibrin-producing hypertropic synovitis. It is conceivable that the remaining fibrin and necrotic tissue may have an unfavourable effect, which is also supported by the positive effect of arthroclysis (joint washings) *(Menkes* et al., *Guaraundon, Isomälk, Collon, Aignan)*. However, only the future and comparable observations of analogous series over a longer time will show us where the safest boundaries lie between the two methods.

5. Discussion

When we survey the results achieved in our knee and finger synovectomy, we can sum up as follows:

1. The vast majority of synovectomy patients have been sick for many years and exhibit a polyarthritic picture and advanced joint changes. Late synovectomies are now undertaken 4 times more than early ones.

2. It is all the more astonishing that even after years, about 3/4 of the cases show a clear improvement in the local disease activity.

3. The improvement concerns primarily the pain and swelling, whereas mobility and deformity are only influenced to an insignificant degree.

4. The X-ray picture hardly changes in the majority of cases. Nevertheless, deteriorations are definitely much more common than improvements. At the same time, we must expect an increase of the secondary osteoarthritic changes, particularly in the case of late synovectomies.

5. There is no satisfactory answer to the question of recurrent synovitis frequency because we have no clear definition or an unbroken serie of biopsy examinations.

6. The general illness and the respective increase in the degree of disability are not influenced to any distinct and appreciably degree by the individual joint synovectomies for a longer time.

7. Chemical and radio-isotope synovectomy warrant more attention. Especially in the case of early synovectomies they are a real alternative to operative synovectomy. Nevertheless, owing to the undisputed advantages, late synovectomies, synovectomy of complex joints (e. g. the wrist) as well as tenosynovectomies still remain, for the present, the principal domain of operative synovectomy.

6. Appendix

| CLINICAL EVALUATION OF RHEUMATOID ARTHRITIS PATIENTS | CLINIK WILH. SCHULTHESS ZÜRICH |

Examiner:

| Last name: | First name: | Birthdate: | Date: |

| Address: | Occupation: | Status no.: |

☐ Righthander   ☐ Lefthander   ☐ male   ☐ female   Patient no.:

Diagnosis: ☐ Juvenile RA   ☐ Seroneg. RA Adult   ☐ Bechterew's Disease
            ☐ Still's Disease   ☐ Special Type RA (Felty etc.)   ☐ Collagenosis
            ☐ Seropos. RA Adult   ☐ Psoriatic Arthritis

Range of Motion (ROM), neutral position = 0
         Method of the American Academy of Orthopedic Surgeons 1965

Code for clinical abnormality (Swanson et al.)

1 thumb swan neck	10 instability	18 rotational deformity
2 thumb boutonniere	11 tendon rupture	19 erosions
3 subluxation-dislocation	12 constrictive tenosynovitis	20 joint narrowing, X-ray
4 swan neck, finger	13 synovial hypertrophy	21 subchondral sclerosis, X-ray
5 boutonniere, finger	14 crepitation with motion	22 painful joint w. motion
6 intrinsic tightness	15 extensor tendon subluxation	23 nerve compression — M.U.R.
7 ulnar drift	16 verus angle	24 vasculitis
8 radial drift	17 valgus angle	25 nodules
9 ankylosis		

Serverity Index   a mild   b moderate   c severe

Activities of Daily Living: I independent   A assisted   U unable

	I	A	U			I	A	U
dressing				hygiene				
upper ext.				hair				
trunk				teeth				
lower ext.				shave				
bath				handwrite				
shower				typewrite				
toilet				telephone				
door-handle				pick up coin				
turn key				eating				
press-stud								

Ambulatory Status   ☐ walking without cane 30 min.   ☐ bicycle yes   ☐ sitting freely
                    ☐ less than 30 min.   ☐ driving yes   ☐ sitting in special chair
                    ☐ walking with 1 cane   ☐ not able to sit
                    ☐ with 2 canes
                    ☐ no walking

Fig. 1 Clinical evaluation of rheumatoid arthritis patients

STATUS OF FINGERS, HANDS, WRISTS

Patient no.: _____

Status no.: _____

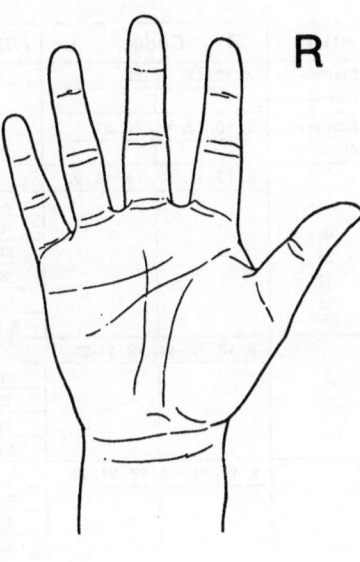

R

Thumb Codes : 1, 2, 3, 9-14, 16, 22							
	R	Codes	L	Joint	R	ROM	L
THUMB				CM Abd			
				CM Add			
				Opp			
				MP			
				IP			
Finger Codes 3-15, 19, 22-25							
INDEX				MP			
				PIP			
				DIP			
	Flex. DIP Crease-Palmar Crease						
MIDDLE				MP			
				PIP			
				DIP			
	Flex. DIP Crease to Palmar Cr.						
RING				MP			
				PIP			
				DIP			
	Flex. DIP Crease-Palamar Crease						
LITTLE				MP			
				PIP			
				DIP			
	Flex. DIP Crease to Palmar Cr.						
Wrist Codes 6, 7-14, 19, 20, 22, 23							
Carpus				Flex			
				Ext			
				U. Drift			
				R. Drift			

GRASP		R	L
CYLINDERS	Diameter		
	2 1/2		
	5		
	7 1/2		
	10		
SPHERES	Diameter		
	5		
	7 1/2		
	10		

Vigorimele

STRENGTH	☐ Atü ☐ Kg/cm ☐ mm Hg		
PULP PINCH	Finger II		
	„ III		
	„ IV		
	„ V		
LATERAL OR KEY PINCH			
GRIP			

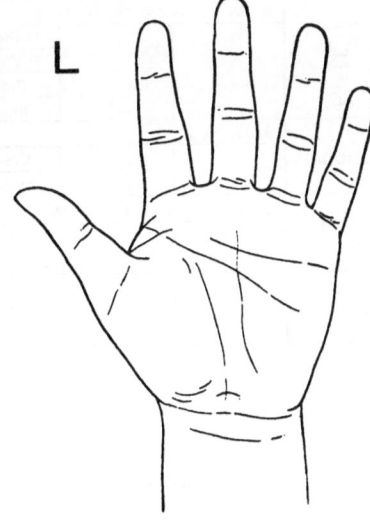

L

STATUS OF OTHER INVOLVED JOINTS

Status no.: _____
Patient no.: _____

JOINT	R	Codes	L	FUNCT.	R	ROM	L
Sterno-clavic.	3, 10, 13, 14, 22						
Acromio-clavic	3, 10, 13, 14, 20, 22						
SHOULDER	9, 10, 11, 13, 14, 19, 22						
SHOULDER				Abd			
SHOULDER				Add			
SHOULDER				Flex			
SHOULDER				Ext			
SHOULDER				J. Rot			
SHOULDER				A. Rot			
ELLBOW	9, 10, 13, 14, 19, 22-25						
ELLBOW				Flex			
ELLBOW				Ext			
ELLBOW				Pro			
ELLBOW				Sup			
HIP	9, 10, 14, 19, 20, 21, 22						
HIP				Flex			
HIP				Ext			
HIP				Abd			
HIP				Add			
HIP				I Rot			
HIP				A Rot			
KNEE	3, 9, 10, 13, 14, 16-21						
KNEE				Flex			
KNEE				Ext			
ANKLE	9, 10, 12, 13, 14, 16, 17, 19, 22						
ANKLE				D. Flex			
ANKLE				P. Flex			
ANKLE				Pro			
ANKLE				Sup			
Chopart	9, 19, 20, 22						
Chopart				Ever			
Chopart				Inver			
GREAT TOE	3, 4, 5, 9, 10, 11, 13, 15, 16, 17						
GREAT TOE				MP			
GREAT TOE				IP			
TOES 2-5				MP			
TOES 2-5				PIP			
TOES 2-5				PIP			

FRONT FOOT

☐ Normal   ☐ Spread foot not contr.   ☐ Spread foot contracted

STATUS OF VERTEBRAL COLUMN

Status no.: _____

Patient no.: _____

	Codes 9, 14, 19, 20, 21, 22, 23	Function	R	ROM	L
CERVICAL VERTEBRAL COLUMN		Rotation Inclin.			
	Chin-Sternum in cm cm	max			
		min			
DORS. VERT. COL.	Dorsal Schober in cm 10/				
LUMBAR VERTEBR. COLUMN	Lumbar Schober in cm 10/				
	Fingertip-floor cm				
Ileo-Sacral					
	Menel's Sign				

PREVIOUS RHEUMATOID SURGERY

Type of Surgery	Date	Pain	Swelling	Deform.	ROM	Funct.	Strength

+ Improvement   ◯ Stationary   — Deterioration

PLANNED RHEUMATOID SURGERY

☐ X-rays
☐ Tomo
☐ Photos
☐ Movies

Signature _____

Bibliography

Aignan, M., M. C. Millet-Tesson, Rheumat. **2**, 149 (1972). – *Allison, N., G. V. Coonse,* Arch. Surg. **18**, 824 (1929). – *Ansell, B. M., O. Crook, J. R. Mellard, G. L. E. Bywaters,* Ann. Rheum. Dis. **22**, 435 (1963). – *Ansell, B. M.,* Ann. rheum. Dis. **32,** 1 (1973). – *Bauer, R., H. Jürger,* Verh. DGOT 57 Kgr. **78** (1971). – *Behnke, H., C. Holland,* Z. Rheumaforschg. **32**, 401 (1973). – *Berglöf, F. E.,* Acta Rheum. Scand. **10**, 92 (1964). – *Boon-Itt, S. B.,* J. Bone J. Surg. **12**, 853 (1930). – *Collan, Y., G. Lorincz, V. Laine,* Scand. J. Rheum. **1**, 27 (1972). – *De la Chapelle, A., M. Oka, A. Rekonen, A. Ruotsi,* Ann. Rheum. Dis. **31**, 508 (1972). – *Delbarre, F., C. J. Menkes, M. Aignan, J. Ingrand, A. Lego, J. C. Roncayrol,* Revue Rhumat. **40**, 205 (1973). – *Delbarre, F.,* Rhumat. **2**, 15 (1972). – *Ellison, M. R., K. J. Kelly, A. E. Flatt,* J. Bone J. Surg. **53-A**, 1041 (1971). – *Fearnley, M. E.,* Ann. Phys. Med. **7**, 294 (1964). – *Fellinger, K., N. Thumb,* Rhumat. **2**, 81 (1972). – *Flatt, A. E.,* Rheumat. **18**, 70 (1962). – *Geens, S., M. L. Clayton, J. D. Leidholt, C. J. Smyth, B. A. Bartholomew,* J. Bone J. Surg. **51-A**, 617 (1969). – *Ghormley, R. K., D. M. Cameron,* Am. J. Surg. **53**, 455 (1941). – *Goldie, J.,* Sem. Arthr. Rheum. **3**, 219 (1974). – *Goldthait, J. E.,* Boston Med. Surg. J. **143**, 286 (1900). – *Gross, D.,* Z. Rheumaforschg. **22**, 456 (1963). – *Guiraudon, C.,* Rhumat. **2**, Suppl. 1, 153 (1972). – *Gumpel, J. M., H. E. Farrar, E. D. Williams,* Ann. Rheum. Dis. **33**, 126 (1974). – *Gumpel, J. M., E. D. Williams, H. Glass,* Rhumat. **2**, 45 (1972). – *Henderson, M. S.,* Surg. Clin. North. Amer. **4**, 565 (1924). – *Hirohata, K., K. Morimoto,* Ultrastructure of Bone and Joint Deseases (Tokyo 1971). – *Isomäki, A. M., H. Inone, M. Oka,* Scand. J. Rheum. **1**, 53 (1972). – *Jakubowski, S.,* pers. Mitteilung. – *Jones, E.,* J. Am. Med. Ass. **81**, 1579 (1923). – *Jaroschy, W.,* Med. Klin. **32**, 1214 (1927). – *Kalliomäki, J. L., S. Jalava, M. Möltönen,* Scand. J. Rheumat. **3**, 25 (1974). – *Kenesi, C.,* Revue Rhumat. **38**, 307 (1971). – *Laine, V., K. Vainio,* Frühsynovektomie bei pcP – Acta rheumatol. Doc. Geigy 25 (Basel 1969). – *Laine, V., K. Vainio,* Z. Rheumaforschg. **29**, 81 (1965). – *Laurin, C. A., J. Desmarchais, L. Daziano, R. Gariepy, A. Derome,* J. Bone J. Surg. **56-A**, 521 (1974). – *Lewis, D. C., M. Ziff,* Arthr. Rheum. **9**, 682 (1966). – *Makin, M., G. C. Robin,* J. Amer. Med. Ass. **188**, 725 (1964). – *Martio, J., H. Isomäki, T. Heikkola, V. Laine,* Scand. J. Rheum. **1**, 5 (1972). – *Mason, R. M.,* Results of Synovectomy of the Knee Joint in Rheumatoid Arthritis. In: Synovectomy and Arthroplasty in RA. (Stuttgart 1967). – *Menkes, C. J., J. P. Allain, C. Gentil, J. Witvoet, H. Tak-Tak, F. Simon, F. Delbarre,* Revue Rhuma. **40**, 255 (1973). – *Menkes, C. J., M. Aignan, B. Galuiche, A. Le Gö,* Rheumat. **2**, 61 (1972). – *Mignon, A.,* Bul. Mem. Soc. Chir. Paris, **26**, 1113 (1900). – *Mohing, W.,* Orthopäde **2**, 75 (1973). – *Mondragon Kalb, M.,* Medicina **15**, 82 (1965). – *Müller, W.,* Arch. f. Klin. Chir. **47**, 1 (1894). – *Murphy, J. B.,* Surg. Clin. Chicago **5**, 155 (1916). – *Niculescu, N.* et al., Z. Rheumaforschg. **29**, 27 (1970). – *Nieny, K.,* Zentr. Bl. f. Chir. **50**, 3218 (1927). – *Oka, M., A. Rekonen, A. Ruotsi,* Acta rheumat. Scand. **6**, 271 (1970). – *Pahle, J.,* Orthopäde **2**, 13 (1973). – *Payr, E.,* Zeitschr. f. Orthop. Chir. **49**, 153 (1927). – *Piattier-Pikatty, C. J. Menkes, J. Juckman, F. Delbarre,* Rhumat. **3**, 65 (1973). – *Von Ries, G., A. Swensson,* Acta Med. Scand. Suppl. **259**, 27 (1951). – *Roberts, S. D., P. J. Gillespie,* Ann. Rheum. Dis. **32**, Suppl. 46 (1973). – *Schüller, M.,* Die Pathologie und Therapie der Gelenkentzündungen. (Wien 1887). – *Speed, J. S.,* J. Am. Med. Assn. **83**, 1814 (1924). – *Steindler, A.,* J. Am. Med. Assn. **84**, 16 (1925). – *Stevenson, A. C.,* Ann. Rheum. Dis. **32**, 19 (1973). – *Sweet, P. P.,* Am. J. Surg. **6**, 807 (1929). – *Taylor, A. R., J. S. Harbison, C. Pepler,* Ann. Rheum. Dis. **31**, 159 (1972). – *Tillmann, K.,* Z. Rheumaforschg. **31**, 278 (1972). – *Tillmann, K.,* Orthopäde **2**, 10 (1973). – *Vainio, K., H. Julkunen,* Acta rheum. Scand. **6**, 25 (1960). – *Virkunen, M., E. E. Krusius, F. Heiskanen,* Acta rheum. Scand. **13**, 81 (1967). – *Volkmann, R.,* Zentr. Bl. f. Chir. **6**, 39 (1977). – *Wilde, A. H., S. R. Sawmiller,* Cleveland Clinic Quart. **36**, 155 (1969). – *Wilde, A. L.,* J. Bone J .Surg. **56-A**, 71 (1974). – *Zuckner, J.* et al., Ann. Rheum. Dis. **25**, 178 (1966).

The influence of knee synovectomy on the course of disease in patients suffering from rheumatoid arthritis (RA)

There is no doubt that RA takes a more favourable course with continuous conservative treatment than with occasional medical supervision. With skilful application of the conservative treatment, the state of health in part of the patients can be kept stable over a longer period. Despite this conservative treatment, however, a number of patients continually experience new episodes of inflammation which can lead to severe disablement of the patient if the disease progresses extremely unfavourably (4,13,18). We endeavour to remedy or reduce disablements occurring in this manner by means of reconstructive surgery (arthrodeses, arthroplasties, reconstructive tendon operations etc.). The decision to undertake such reconstructive operations as well as the evaluation of the respective operation results are left exclusively to the operating surgeon because such operations are limited to local corrections (16). Synovectomies are quite different. The introduction of synovectomy in the treatment programme for RA patients has opened the way for new expectations. Apart from the purely local treatment, they also concern the general therapeutic and preventive possibilities. To clarify the question of the preventive and general therapeutic effects of synovectomy, it is necessary for the rheumatologist and the surgeon to cooperate closely. In contrast to reconstructive operations, it is important for both of them to agree on the patients selected for operation and the time it should be carried out. This also applies to the post-operative treatment and the evaluation of the immediate and long-term results.

Examination methods and patient material

With a view to meeting this pre-requisite, we prepared a project for a joint surgical-rheumatological study in 1967. An examination calender was included in this study. It provided for a pre-examination (at the earliest 30 days before the operation) and three examinations in the first year after the operation (3, 6 and 12 months after the synovectomy) and finally a yearly check. The examination results were recorded on ready-prepared questionaires. The entries related to the anamnestic, clinical and therapeutica-data, as well as the biohumoral, immunoserological, histological and roentgenological findings (Fig. 18 – Layout of the questionaire). The surgical part of the work shows how the documentation was kept for the joint to be operated or the actually operated joint. All the examinations were carried out by a rheumatologist in order to exclude any possible – even if unintended – subjectivity (of the operating surgeon). Since the following part of the study only concerns itself with the synovectomy problems from the rheumatological standpoint, only the results of the knee synovectomies are considered. They are best suited for a study of this kind.

The work endeavours to answer two problem circles, namely:

1. Whether the synovectomy result is dependent on the pre-operative disease state as well as the biohumoral and/or immunoserological disease activity.

2. Whether the synovectomy can check the progress of the disease or slow it down to a noticeable degree, as well as retard the biohumoral and/or immunoserological activity.

The following assessment criteria were laid down in order to answer these questions:

a) For the progress of the disease: the respective state of illness according to *Steinbrocker*.

b) For the biohumoral disease activity: the sedimentation rate, leukocytes and serum iron content of the patient's blood.

c) For the immunoserological disease activity: the rheumatoid factors of the patient's blood.

Fig. 18 Layout of the questionaire

Sex, age

A. General

1. Hereditary trait, 2. Previous trauma or illness, 3. Beginning of RA, 4. Joint involvement, 5. Type of affliction, 6. Duration of disease, 7. Stage of RA, 8. Degree of function.

B. Previous treatment

I General

1. Salicylates, 2. Gold salts, 3. Anti-malarials, 4. Corticosteroids, 5. Antimetabolites, 6. Penicillinamine, 7. Pyrazolon, 8. Indomethacin, 9. Other medicines, 10. i.a. steroids, 11. Thiotepa i.a., 12. Phys. therapy, 13. Radiotherapy, 14. Previosly conducted synovectomy.

II Local (joint intended for operation)

15. i.a. Steriods, 16. i.a. Thiotepa, 17. Intra-articular application of other drugs involvement

C. Joint status (joint intended for operation)

I Clinical findings

1. Spontaneous pain, 2. Tenderness pain under the application of pressure, 3. Overheating, 4. Swelling, 5. Effusion, 6. Thickening of the capsule, 7. Muscular atrophy, 8. Rheumatoid nodules, 9. Deformation, 10. Movement, 11. Grip-strength

II X-ray findings

12. Osteoporosis, 13. Soft tissue swellung, 14. Interarticular space, 15. Erosions, 16. subchondral cysts, 17. Deformation

D. Laboratory findings

I General

1. Sed. rate, 2. Hb, 3. Erthrocytes, 4. Leukocytes, 5. Electrophoresis, 6. Serum iron, 7. Serum copper, 8. Blood sugar, 9. Cholesterin, 10. Urea, 11. Creatinine, 12. Uric acid, 13. Transaminases, 14. Bilirubin, 15. Calcium, 16. Alkal. phosphatase, 17. Urine

II Rheumatoid factors (Rf)

18. ELF, 19. Singer-Plotz, 20. Waaler-Rose, 21. antiglobulin consumption test latex slide destillieous latex test according to, 22. LE phenomenon, 23. Complementary titer Hemolytic complement

III Immunologic findings in synovial fluid

24. Singer-Plotz test, 25. Waaler-Rose test, 26. Rf in leukocytehomogenate, 27. Rhagocytes, 28. Hemolytic gomplementaty complement

We have not undertaken a detailed comparison of many of the biochemical findings (mentioned in table 18) prior to and after synovectomy During the course of the study it was found that the findings were not particularly conclusive. For the same reasons, we have not evaluated the hemolytic complement in the patient's serum. Originally, they were were regarded as the second (besides the rheumatoid factor) assessment criterion for the immunoserological disease activity.

102 knee synovectomies performed on 72 pcP patients (60 women and 12 men) were evaluated. The data for the patients' ages, duration of illness, as well as the stage of illness prior to the synovectomy are summarized in Figs. 19, 20 and 21.

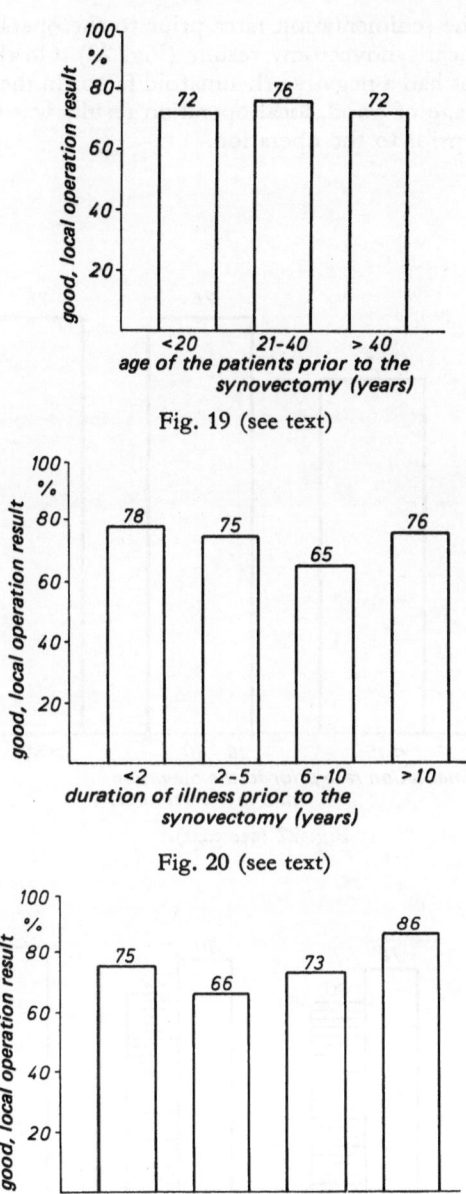

Fig. 19 (see text)

Fig. 20 (see text)

Fig. 21 (see text)

Synovectomy results

The percentage of good, local operation results was not dependent on the age of the patients, the duration of the illness or the pre-operation stage of illness.

The behaviour of the sedimentation rates prior to the operation also showed no influence on the local synovectomy results (Fig. 22). On the other hand, in the case of patients that had a negative rheumatoid factor in the blood before the operation, the percentage of good, local operation results was higher than those where it was positive prior to the operation.

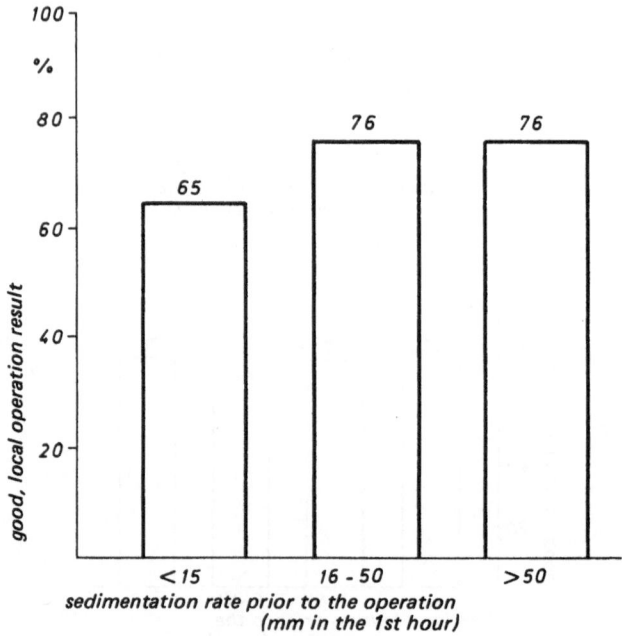

Fig. 22 (see text)

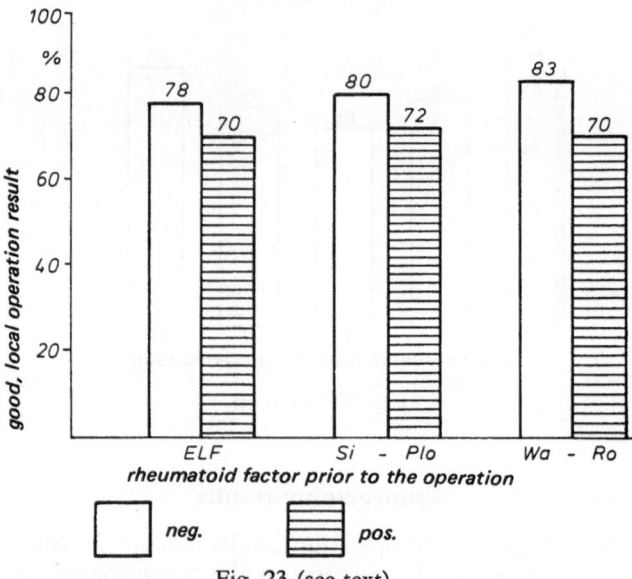

Fig. 23 (see text)

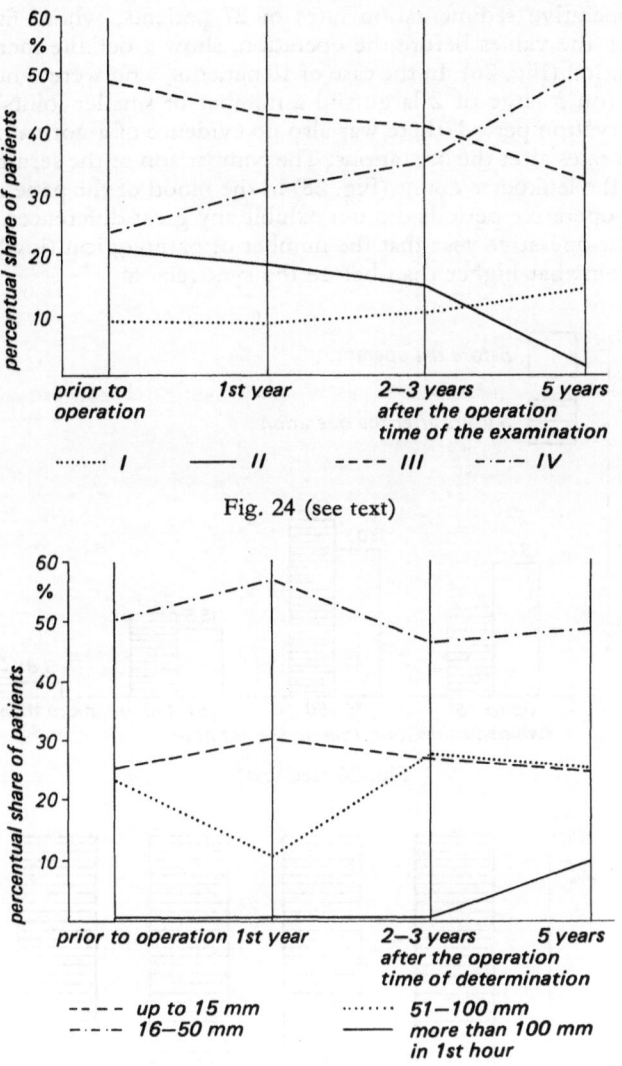

Fig. 24 (see text)

Fig. 25 (see text)

The percentage of patients in illness stage I remained constant throughout the entire post-operative observation period (up to the fifth year after the synovectomy). However, the percentage of patients in stages 2 and 3 has definitely declined. At the same time, the percentage of patients in stage 4 is twice as large in the 5th post-operative year than before the synovectomy (Fig. 24). The sedimentation rates show slight fluctuations in the post-operative period. In the first post-operative year, they were somewhat lower in the case of patients with higher values (51–100 mm/h) than before the operation. Two to three and five years after the synovectomy they were the same again as before the operation (Fig. 25).

The post-operative sedimentation rates of 27 patients, whose findings were compared with the values before the operation, show a definite increase 5 years after the operation (Fig. 26). In the case of 10 patients, who were synovectomized several times (on 3 large or 2 large and a number of smaller joints) during the five-year observation period, there was also no evidence of a normalization in the sedimentation rates after the operations. The comparison of the serum iron values (Fig. 27) and the leukocyte count (Fig. 28) in the blood of the patient during the pre- and post-operative periods did not exhibit any great differences. It was only in the first post-operative year that the number of pathological (low) serum iron values were somwhat higher than before the synovectomy.

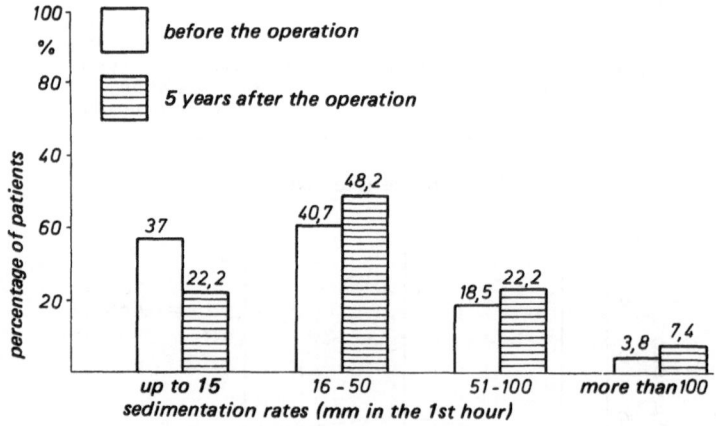

Fig. 26 (see text)

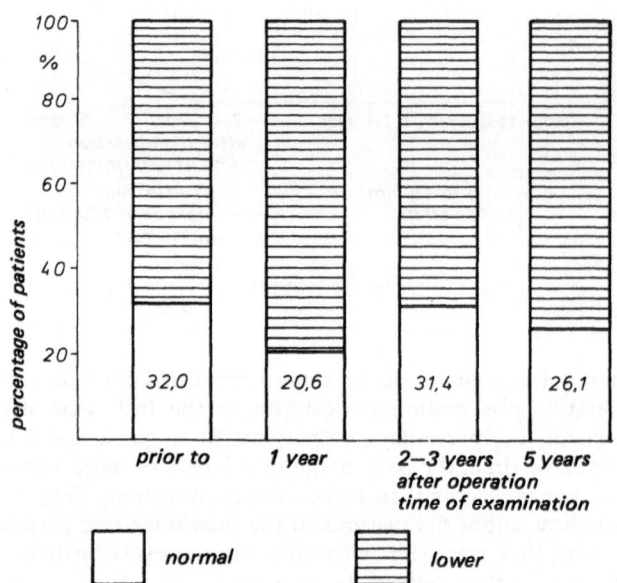

Fig. 27 (see text)

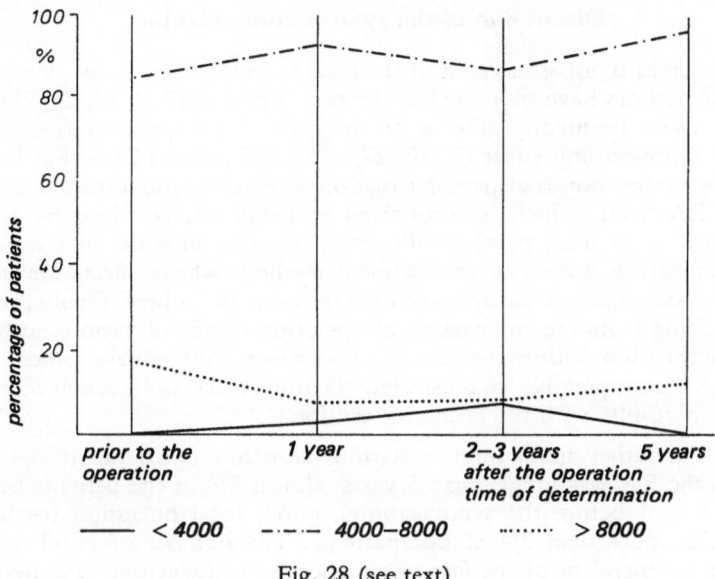

Fig. 28 (see text)

On the other hand, the number of patients with positive rheumatoid factors in the blood, as well as two to three years after the synovectomy was less than before the operation (valid for all three methods used to determine the rheumatoid factor) The difference was statistically significant for the *Singer-Plotz* test (p — 0.05). However, five years after the operation the number of patients with postive rheumatoid factors had increased to such an extent that their percentage was greater than before the synovectomy (Fig. 29). With the 10 patients that had been synovectomized several times it was established that the rheumatoid factors in the blood were seven and five times positive before and after the opertaions respectively.

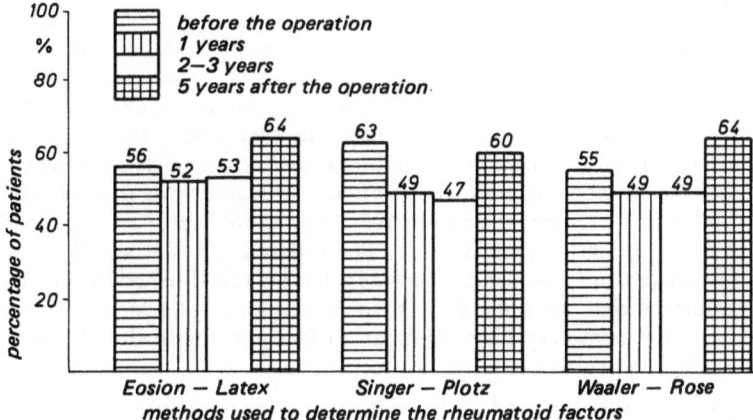

Fig. 29 (see text)

Discussion of the synovectomy results

When it comes to an assessment of the local synovectomy results, we find that most of the authors have more or less the same opinion (2, 9, 19, 20, 21). However, their views frequently differ as to the general therapeutical as well as the preventive synovectomy effect (7, 10, 27). This difference of opinion is chiefly attributable to the non-transparent situation after the synovectomy. Even the course of RA itself, which is recognized as being characterized by surprises (spontaneous remissions, psychic influences, etc.) provides the first difficulties. The post-operative, conservative treatment method, whose effects are not easy to separate from those of the synovectomy, provide the others. Finally, the difficulties resulting from the comparison of operation results of various authors are also significant (non-uniform periods of observation, different assessment criteria etc.) (8, 16). Consequently, we must view the preventive and general therapeutic synovectomy results with the necessary caution.

Despite the rather unfavourable starting situation (with nearly 3/4 of the operations the RA was longer than 5 years, almost 3/4 of the patients belonged to stages 3 or 4 before the synovectomy), good, local operation results were attained with more than 3/4 of our patients. The number of good operation results was independent of the fact of whether the synovectomy was performed on younger or older patients, after a shorter or longer period of illness, as well as whether it was carried out in the beginning or advanced stage of the RA. *Jakubowski* (20), *Mohing* (23), *Danielisz* (9), *Barbier* (2) and other authors (8, 18) have been able to report similar successes with knee synovectomy. *Goldie* and *Schlossmann* (15), as well as *McEven* (22), have purposely investigated the dependency of the synovectomy results on the preoperative illness stages of the RA patients. In this respect, they have not found any dependency.

On the other hand, *Gariepy* (14) has established this. His good operation results (79% with 56 patients) may be related exclusively to the early synovectomies (stages 2 and 3). With the late synovectomies (stages 3 and 4), he experienced only failures. *Hertel* (19) saw an unsatisfactory synovectomy result in 70% of the cases following a late synovectomy. In the opinion of *Barnes* (3) if the joint to be operated has been afflicted for more than five years, it constitutes a contra-indication to synovectomy.

The number of good, local synovectomy results was not dependent on the pre-operative sedimentation rates in the case of our patients. *Vainio* (26), *Mason* (21), as well as *Morgan* and his colleagues (24) also found no relevant dependency. *Arden* (1) and *Drablos* (11), however, maintain that good, local synovectomy results are seldom found when the biohumoral disease activity is extensive. With our patients, the number of good, local operation results was greater where the patients exhibited a pre-operative negative rheumatoid factor in the blood than those with a pre-operative positive one. The difference is statistically significant for the *Singer-Plotz* test (p — 0.005). *Barnes* (3) has also established this dependency He also maintains that we must expect, in principle, poor synovectomy results with patients that have very high rheumatoid factor titres in the blood. *Drablos* dismisses such a dependency.

The majority of the operated patients in stage 1 of the illness belonged to the same stage five years after the synovectomy. However, over the same period a considerable number of the late synovectomies (stages 2 and 3) had to be classified under a higher stage. The results show that we may expect a certain preventive operational effect with the early synovectomies. To what extent the post-operative conservative treatment has played a part in these results cannot be answered conclusively. It was continued post-operatively for patients of all disease stages, exactly in the same way as for the non-operated RA patients. For ethical reasons, we were not allowed to form so-called control groups.

Analogously, *Dupont* (12) and other authors (2, 18, 20 and 26) confirm that improvement is likely to last longer with early synovectomies than with later ones.

In the case of our patients, we did not find that the operation has a continuous effect on the sedimentation rate. Although a certain downward trend was established among the patients with high sedimentation rates (51–100 mm/h) in the first post-operative year, it could not be determined in the second to third and the fifth post-operative year. Similar results are shown by other supplementary examinations. With 27 patients – where a comparison was made of the pre- and post-operative sedimentation rates, the post-operative figure was clearly higher than the pre-operative five years after the operation. The influence of the synovectomy on the behaviour of the sedimentation rate is assessed differently by the various authors. For example, *Vainio* (26), *Franke* (13) and *Mohing* (23) report a downward trend. Nevertheless, the examinations made by these authors only covered a short period of observation, at the most one year. Under these conditions (downward trend only, limited short period only), these results line up with ours. On the other hand, *Crasselt* and *Schedwill* (8) report a significant decrease in the sedimentation rates during the first post-operative year. *Mason* (21) and *Drablos* (11) claim that the post-operative sedimentation rates before the synovectomy were higher with some of the patients and lower in others.

The leukocyte and serum iron values – our other two assessment criteria for the biohumoral disease activity – show no tendency to decline in the post-operative period. We were unable to find any comparable data in the literature. *Crasselt* and *Schedwill* (8), however, have included another assessment criterion for biohumoral disease activity in their examinations. On the basis of the behaviour of the C-reactive proteins (CRP), they feel that the downward trend of the biohumoral disease activity is confirmed.

The percentage of our patients with positive rheumatoid factors in the blood was smaller, as well as two to three years after the synovectomy than before the operation. In the fifth post-operative year, the percentage of patients with a positive rheumatoid factor was higher than pre-operative. It was only after repeated synovectomies that the percentage of patients with positive rheumatoid factors was smaller in the fifth post-operative year than in the period prior to the operation. This result would appear to confirm the assumption that the immuno-serological activity of the RA can be retarded for a specific period if correspondingly large portions of the pathologically changed synovial membrane can be removed. The rheumatoid factors formed in the synovial membrane probably play an important role in the immunoserological overall activity. Whereas *Crasselt* and *Schedwill* (8) have established a reduction of the rheumatoid factor titre after the operation in 50% of the patients, they were unable to detect an increase in the titre with any of their patients. *Panova* and *Buchtojarowe* (25) also report a decline in the immunoserological disease activity following a synovectomy. On the other hand, *Craechiolo* and *Bernett* (7) did not establish any significant displacement of the rheumatoid factor titre in connection with the synovectomies.

We cannot make any conclusive statements in respect of the rheumatoid factor titre in the joint-puncture fluids on the basis of our observations (recurring effusion; in some cases pre-operative negative rheumatoid serology was indicated). *Chrachiolo* and *Bernett* (7) report a significant reduction (4 titre stages) in the rheumatoid factor in the joint-pressure fluids of RA patients after synovectomy (in 11 of 21 patients). However, these results may be attributed to two different reasons. They could indicate a production retardation of the rheumatoid factors (elimination of one of the rheumatoid factor production sources) or that no real recurrent synovitis is present. *Gschwend* (16) draws attention to the fact that in the post-operative period a part of the joint-puncture fluid has the character of a recurring effusion, as is found in the case of degenerative joint changes. Such joint effusions can occur in the post-operative period with previously existing (or rapidly developing) gonarthrosis, and only indicate an activation of the degenerative joint process. Such joint effusions are also found with the instability of joints, chondromalacia, etc. (concomitant) of the RA in the advanced stage.

To sum up, it may be said that the patients' ages, the duration of illness and the stage of illness all had no decisive effect on the number of good, local results obtained with knee synovectomies. The synovectomy results were also independent of the pre-operative biohumoral disease activity (as a result of the behaviour of the sedimentation rates, leukocyte and serum iron values measured in the patients' blood). In the case of patients with pre-operative negative rheumatoid factors in the blood, the success quota for the knee synovectomies was higher than with patients whose pre-operative rheumatoid serology was positive.

With patients that were able to be synovectomized in the initial stage (Stage 1), we were able to establish indication of a preventive operative effect. The late synovectomies have not been able to check the progress of the disease. The biohumoral disease activity could not be influenced by the knee synovectomy. Neither early nor late synovectomies have shown differences in this respect. The knee synovectomies appear to be able to retard the immunoserological disease activity for a certain period of time. The degree and duration of influence probably depend – among other things – on the quantity of pathologically changed synovial membrane removed.

Summary

The results are based on 102 knee synovectomies performed on 72 RA patients. The period of observation was five years. The clinical, biohumoral, immunoserological and other parameters were investigated prior to the operation and at yearly intervals after the synovectomy, and the findings noted in ready-prepared questionaires. The respective state of the disease according to the *Steinbrocker* criteria, as well as the actual bihumoral (sedimentation rate, leukocytes and serum iron content of the patients' blood) and the immunoserological (rheumatoid factors in the serum) disease activity were then used as a basis to establish, on the one hand, the dependency of good local results on the pre-operative state of the patient and, on the other, to determine the influence of the synovectomy on the post-operative course of the disease. As a result of this, we were able to establish the following:

1. The pre-operative sero-negative patients exhibited better local operation results than their sero-positive counterparts.

2. The progress of RA was able to be checked during the five-year study period with the majority of patients synovectomized in Stage 1.

3. In a number of patients, the immonuserological disease activity could be retarded for a longer period of time (2 to 3 years) as a result of the knee synovectomy.

Bibliography

1. *Arden, G. P.*, The results of synovectomy in rheumatoid arthritis. *Chapchal, G.*, Synovectomy and arthroplasty in rheumatoid arthritis – 2nd Internat. Symp. 1967 Basle, Switzerland, 83 (Stuttgart 1967). – 2. *Barbier, M.*, Die Synovektomie in der Behandlung der pcP, Ergebnisse bei 100 Kniegelenk- und 300 Fingergelenksynovektomien. Inaugural-Dissertation Universität (Zürich 1972). – 3. *Barnes, C. G.*, Indications and contraindications for synovectomy of the knee joint in rheumatoid arthritis. *Chapchal, G.*, Synovectomy and arthroplasty in rheumatoid arthritis – 2nd Internat. Sympos. 1967 (Basle, Switzerland) 26 (Stuttgart 1967). – 4. *Böni, A.*, Therapwoch. **20**, 17, 708 (1970). – 5. *Branemark, P. J., R. Ekholm, J. Goldic, J. Lindström*, Acta Rheum. Scand. **13**, 161–189 (1967). – 6. *Cech, O., F. Stryhal*, Synovectomy of the knee joint in rheumatoid arthritis. *Chapchal, G.*, Synovectomy and arthroplasty in rheumatoid arthritis – 2nd Internat. Symp. 1967 (Basle, Switzerland) 35 (Stuttgart 1967). – 7. *Carcchiolo, A., E. V. Bernett*, Arthr. Rheum. **12**, 415 (1969). – 8. *Crasselt, C., K. Schedwill*, Z. Rheumaforschg. **30**, 10–118 (1971). – 9. *Danielisz, L.*, Aeta Arthop. Belg. **63**, 58 (1972). – 10. *De Sèze, S., J. Debeyre, N. Debeyre, J. Couchet*, Rev. Rhum. **34**, 7–8 (416–429), (1967). – 11. *Drabløs, P. A.*, Scand. J. Rheumat. **1**, 49 (1972). – 12. *Dupont, M.*, Acta orthop. belg. **33**, 389–510 (1967). – 13. *Franke, M.*, Therapwoch. **37**, 3212–3219 (1973). – 14. *Gariépy, R.*, The prophylactic effect of synovectomy of the knee in rheumatoid arthritis. *Chapchal, G.*, Synovectomy and arthroplasty in rheumatoid arthritis – 2nd Internat. Symp. 1967 (Basle, Switzerland) 55 (Stuttgart 1967). – 15. *Goldie, J., D. Schlossmann*, Clinical Orthop. and related research **64**, 98 (1969). – 16. *Gschwend, N.*, Die operative Behandlung der progressiv chronischen Polyarthritis (Stuttgart 1968). – 17. *Gschwend, N.*, Präventive Operationen bei pcP (Synovektomien). Die primär chronische Polyarthritis Diagnose und Therapie, Hrsg. *R. Bauer* (Stuttgart 1973). – 18. *Gschwend, N., J. Winer, A. Böni*, Therap. Umschau **31**, 475 (1974). – 19. *Hertel, E.*, Orth. Grenzgeb. **608** (1971). – 20. *Jakubowski, S.*, Rehabilitation of the operated knee-joint. *Chapchal, G.*, Synovectomy and arthroplasty in rheumatoid arthritis – 2nd Internat. Symp. 1967 (Basle, Switzerland) 59 (Stuttgart 1967). – 21. *Mason, R. M.*, Results of synovectomy of the knee joint in rheumatoid arthritis. *Chapchal, G.*, Synovectomy and arthroplasty in rheumatoid arthritis – 2nd Internat. Symp. 1967 (Basle, Switzerland) 47 (Stuttgart 1967). – 22. *Mc Ewen, C.*, New Engl. J. Med. **279**/8 (420–422), (1968). – 23. *Mohing, W.*, Deutsch. Med. Wochschr. **43**, 1961 (1967). – 24. *Morgan, E. S., W. M. Boger, B. C. Gilliland, S. Meyerowitz*, Arthr. and Rheumat. **13**, 761 (1970). – 25. *Panova, M. J., F. E. Buchtojarowa*, The results of synovectomy of the knee joint in various stages of rheumatoid arthritis. *Chapchal, G.*, Synovectomy and arthroplasty in rheumatoid arthritis – 2nd Internat. Symp. 1967 (Basle, Switzerland) 53 (Stuttgart 1967). – 26. *Vainio, K.*, Rheumatism **22**, 10 (1967). – 27. *Winer, J., A. Böni, W. Busse*, Medecine et Hygiène **30**, 1959–1961 (1972).

Der Rheumatismus

Herausgegeben von Prof. Dr. Dr. RUDOLF SCHOEN (Göttingen)

Bezieher der Zeitschrift für Rheumatologie erhalten 20% Nachlaß.

DR. DIETRICH STEINKOPFF VERLAG · DARMSTADT